T0210793

# FROM PATHOLOGY TO POLITICS

# FROM PATHOLOGY TO POLITICS

## PUBLIC HEALTH IN AMERICA

# JAMES T. BENNETT AND THOMAS J. DiLORENZO

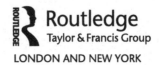

Routledge
Taylor & Francis Group

LONDON AND NEW YORK

First published 2000 by Transaction Publishers

Published 2017 by Routledge
4 Park Square, Milton Park, Abingdon, Oxon OX14 4RN
605 Third Avenue, New York, NY 10017

*Routledge is an imprint of the Taylor & Francis Group, an informa business*

Library of Congress Catalog Number: 00-030270

Library of Congress Cataloging-in-Publication Data
Bennett, James T.
    From pathology to politics: public health in America / James T. Bennett, Thomas J. DiLorenzo.
        p. cm.
    Includes bibliographical references and index.
    ISBN 0-7658-0023-3 (alk. paper)
        1.  Public health—United States-History.  2.  Public health—Social aspects—United States—History.  I. DiLorenzo, Thomas J.  II.  Title.

RA445 .B45  2000
362. 1'0973—dc21                                                    00-030270


ISBN 13: 978-1-4128-0736-4 (pbk)
ISBN 13: 978-0-7658-0023-7 (hbk)

# Contents

# Acknowledgements

*From Pathology to Politics: Public Health in America* is our third book to appear under the auspices of Transaction Publishers. Our two earlier volumes, *CancerScam: Diversion of Federal Funds to Politics* (1998) and *The Food and Drink Police: America's Nannies, Busybodies, and Petty Tyrants* (1999), set the stage for the central topic explored in this current work: the disturbing trend in contemporary American society toward the politicization of health. One would think that most health issues are beyond the pale of the political arena; after all, politics can hardly cure disease or halt epidemics.

We believe that an insidious agenda is being pursued in the name of public health — the use of the coercive power of the state by special interest groups who use health issues for two broad purposes. First, public health matters are a smoke screen to camouflage self-interested behavior, or what economists call "rent seeking." Put simply, health activists lobby for legislation (primarily tax increases that are "earmarked" for their particular causes) and regulations at all levels of government that benefit them financially. Second, health issues are used to advance an ideological agenda — an agenda which, without exception, fosters an enhanced role for the state in every aspect of our lives and in our lifestyles. Some of the initiatives advocated by Those Who Know Best are actually harmful to public health.

We thank the Sunmark Foundation for generous research support that made this book possible and the Locke Institute; excellent research assistance was provided by Matthias Eng, Christopher Farris, and Matthew Tedeschi. We alone are responsible for any errors.

# 1

# Introduction

> *"It began as one man's search for the cause of cholera. It
> has grown into a global response to the devastating effects
> of violence, pollution, poverty and urban decay; to the
> consequences of the suppression of human rights; to alcohol
> and tobacco addiction; and to the spread of AIDS."*
>
> — *Robin Marantz Henig,* The People's Health

Almost daily the American media broadcast news of the latest public health threat. Some of us are told that we may live in a "cancer cluster" — an area with a disproportionate number of cancer deaths — and worry ourselves sick over it. Those of us who live in or near urban areas are informed daily during the summer months about smog measurements and air pollution alerts and are told to stay inside, refrain from exercise, and avoid breathing the outside air, if possible. City water supplies are frequently accused of being health hazards, and at times it seems as though virtually everything we eat and drink is touted by some "public health expert" as being bad for us.

Our homes are said to be filled with "indoor air pollution"; our cars burn too much gasoline (Vice President Gore advocates the elimination of the internal combustion engine[1]); we own too many firearms; we fail to teach our children proper eating, drinking, and lifestyle habits; we are too fat; and some of us are too skinny.

Or so we are told by numerous public health professionals employed by federal, state, and local governments, schools of public health within the nation's universities, health charities, and elsewhere. Granted, life is full of peril and there are indeed genuine public health crises, such as the AIDS epidemic. But to put all this into perspective, it should be noted that Americans are living longer today than they ever have before. As a society, we are as healthy as we have ever been. Why, then, the almost daily announcements of new public health threats and proclamations of impending crises?

1

This is one of the questions that we address in this book. We do not deny that the public health profession, which is comprised of thousands of health researchers, educators, sanitation and pollution control experts, nurses, physicians, and other health care professionals, have made (and continue to make) significant contributions to improving the public's health. As described in chapter 2, the public health movement of the late nineteenth and early twentieth centuries prolonged and saved millions of lives by discovering cures for such deadly diseases as cholera and yellow fever and by pioneering the science of sanitation, among other things.

But the economic law of diminishing returns applies to public health as much as it does to everything else. That is, in the early days of the public health movement each million dollars spent inoculating the public against disease, improving sanitation, and cleaning the air and water, and so on, produced sizable public health benefits. But today each dollar spent on public health expenditures (mostly by federal, state, and local governments) seems to buy much less in terms of improving the quality of life or extending it. We are still benefiting enormously from the advances of the past, but each new public health "advance" no longer produces the dramatic effects that it might have 100 years ago.

In the meantime, a large public health bureaucracy has been created, mostly in the form of federal, state, and local government public health officials; the faculty and administrators of schools of public health at the nation's universities; the executive and staff of various health charities; and nurses, physicians, and other health professionals. This public health bureaucracy is made up of many conscientious, hard-working, dedicated professionals who have devoted their careers to improving children's health, searching for cures to diseases, educating the public on healthy lifestyles, helping us make life less risky, and myriad other good causes. But, as a movement, today's public health profession sometimes seems too preoccupied with expanding governmental programs that would require employing additional public health professionals, even if the likely public health benefits of the program are negligible or nonexistent. This is another major theme of this book: The public health bureaucracy, like all bureaucracies, is concerned with expanding its own size, scope, and budgets, even when such an expansion provides nebulous benefits to the public.

Another thrust of our analysis is that, like all government-funded bureaucracies, the public health bureaucracy has become politicized. Politicization, per se, is not unequivocally bad. One can argue that lobbying efforts by the public health establishment for improved funding of urban sanitation, for example, provided significant benefits to society. But we demonstrate in later chapters that the *leaders* of the American public health movement — the people who run the American Public Health Association, the senior faculty and administrators of schools of public health, many health charity executives, and federal, state, and local government public health officials — are excessively concerned with political issues that too often seem to have little to do with improving public health. The American Public Health Association — the trade association of the public health movement — has used its resources to develop a platform for the promotion of government-controlled medical care, the abolition of the Second Amendment to the U.S. Constitution, a governmental takeover of child care, an expansion of government's role in economic "planning," and other social and economic issues. As this chapter's epigraph states, the public health movement is no longer interested primarily in the eradication of disease; it claims to offer expertise on virtually every social issue, from poverty to human rights.

Chapter 2 traces the history and evolution of the American public health movement from its founding, right after the Civil War, until the 1950s. This was the period of great advances in public health in the form of the eradication of deadly diseases, vast improvements in sanitation and hygiene, and lengthened life expectancy. During this period a public health "infrastructure" was created in the form of public health departments in local governments across the United States, along with other public health institutions at the state and federal levels of government, such as the Public Health Service, the federal Department of Health and Human Services, the National Institutes of Health, and the federal Centers for Disease Control.

Chapter 3 describes a transformation in public health that occurred during the 1960s that falls under the rubric of the "new" public health. Beginning in the mid-1960s the public health establishment began to change its focus from the eradication of disease to social policy. Public health professionals began pursuing education in such fields as sociology, anthropology, and political science, as opposed to such traditional public health fields of medicine, sanitary science, chemistry, physiology, pathology, and bacteriology. Consequently, the modern public health professional is as likely to consider herself a political activist as a medical problem solver.

Chapter 4 catalogues the "radicalization" of the public health movement by discussing how its numerous political initiatives seem to have little to do with directly improving public health or, in some cases, are even likely to be harmful to it. For example, during the Cold War the American Public Health Association issued numerous statements supporting communist governments all over the world. The APHA seems especially proud of Cuba and, during the 1980s, was a champion of the communist regime in Nicaragua, ostensibly because these two dictatorships seized control of their countries' health care systems along the lines the APHA would like to see adopted in the U.S.

The APHA persistently condemns the profit motive, competition, and the institutions of capitalism with regard to the provision of health care. We question the ability of government-controlled medical care to improve the nation's health, based on the experiences in other countries, such as England and Canada.

Chapters 5 through 9 are case studies of the politicization of the public health movement in America. Chapter 5 discusses how the public health movement is at the forefront of the political movement to dilute, if not repeal, the Second Amendment right to bear arms by defining violence as a "public health" problem. One feature of the public health movement's crusade against the Second Amendment is a long list of dubious "research" articles on the alleged dangers of gun ownership that we show are seriously flawed.

Chapter 6 is a case study of the political approach to public health problems that is increasingly adopted by public health professionals. Once a public health problem, such as smoking, is chosen, the public health movement increasingly advocates prohibition as its preferred "solution." No one denies that smoking is a health hazard. But most Americans are also aware that prohibition, like that of alcohol in the 1920s and 1930s, was a debacle. Nevertheless, the approach to the problem of smoking-related diseases preferred by public health professionals is what one might call creeping prohibitionism — to lobby the government to impose higher taxes on the "undesirable" behavior, such as smoking, and then earmark some of the tax revenues *to the public health professionals and their organizations* to be used to finance additional lobbying efforts for even higher taxes, constitutionally dubious advertising bans, or outright prohibition. This is the modus operandi that the public health movement adopted in the war against smoking and which is now, as we write, being employed in the movement against gun ownership and alcohol consumption. It is likely that the same kinds of political crusades will be launched in the near future against other "politically incorrect" products, such as fast food, beef, soft drinks, caffeine, and automobiles.[2]

Chapter 7, "Nothing But Politics," shows just how politically oriented the public health movement has become by surveying the APHA's various announcements and activities with regard to various social and economic issues. One gets the distinct impression in reading the APHA literature that politics is the *central* focus of the organization and that the direct improvement of public health, for some health professionals, is only a secondary concern.

Chapter 8 discusses the politicization of public health "science." Although there is much excellent research performed by public health researchers at universities, governmental institutions, and nonprofit organizations, there is also a lot of "political science" in the public health movement. This chapter reveals the various methods of statistical manipulation that are used by certain public health researchers to "cook the data" in order to achieve politically correct results. For example, many of the almost daily findings of "cancer clusters" and other alleged dangers are often mere statistical illusions created by government-funded researchers who are under intense pressure to "verify" preconceived research "results." The result is what one might call public health "disease mongering."

Chapter 9 discusses the disturbing phenomenon of the public health movement's crusade to effectively place the child care industry in America under government control. Institutionalized child care has many flaws, such as the impossibility of providing children with needed individual attention and the proliferation of diseases in most child care centers. These problems are likely to be amplified if the industry were to be nationalized.

The tenth and final chapter contains a brief summary of the main themes of the book and discusses the implications of the transformation of public health from pathology to politics.

# 2

## History and Evolution of the
## American Public Health Movement

*"Americans are not dying the way they once did."*
— *Jacob Sullum,* For Your Own Good[1]

Of the 620,000 battle-related deaths during the War Between the States, fewer than half of them were caused by wounds; disease accounted for the rest. In the 1860s there was virtually no knowledge of sanitation, bacteriology, and germs. Battlefield surgeons routinely cleaned their surgical tools with dirty rags or washed them in river or rain water before performing the next operation. Because tens of thousands of men were forced to live in very close quarters during the war, thousands of soldiers perished from epidemics of yellow fever, small-pox, cholera, typhoid, and typhus, among other diseases. When the war ended and the soldiers returned home, they sometimes started disease epidemics throughout the country.

A New York City physician described the city in 1860 as a "fever nest" where, in one tenement house he entered, "the doors and windows were broken, the cellar was filled with sewage, every room was occupied by families of Irish immigrants who had but little furniture and slept on straw scattered on the floor."[2] In 1865 there was no sanitary administration at all in New York City or in most other cities.

The first governmental health department devoted to improving sanitation and controlling communicable diseases was started in Massachusetts in 1869 — four years after the war. The Massachusetts Health Department focused on medical education, sanitation, disease research, enforcing quarantines, and cooperating with newly created local-government health departments. This would become the model for state and local government public health initiatives.

The creation of government health departments — empowered to administer inoculations, regulate sanitary conditions, and to try to eradicate various diseases (e.g., by controlling mosquitoes) — is said to be a response to a "free-rider" problem. (Because everyone receives the benefit of insect control whether she pays for it or not, no one has an incentive to pay, i.e., all wish to "ride free.") Controlling communicable disease generates benefits that all citizens enjoy, although it is difficult, if not impossible, to get individual citizens to pay for those benefits voluntarily. Especially in larger communities, such as a larger city, there is the inevitable temptation to "free ride"— to let others pay for the public good. The problem is that if enough people think this way, the public good will either not be provided, or it will be provided in insufficient quantities. Thus, this "public goods problem" becomes the rationale for government intervention in public health. Control of communicable disease and health-related research was performed for public benefit.

The early boards of health concentrated on improving sanitation and enforcing ordinances regarding waste disposal, street drainage, removal of filth, drainage of swamps, and, later, immunizations, and quarantines of homes and ships.[3] By 1890 every state had a board of health, and there were hundreds of local boards.

Public health was greatly improved in the postwar years by numerous scientific discoveries as well. Antiseptic surgery was developed in 1869 by British surgeon Joseph Lister, a student of Louis Pasteur, the chemist and microbiologist who developed the process of "pasteurization" in the 1860s. Pasteur's work led to the creation of the field of bacteriology. Pasteur discovered the pneumococcus, the bacillus of malignant edema, and the germ of chicken cholera, for which he developed a vaccine in 1881. He also developed a vaccination against anthrax in that year, while others discovered staphylococcus and streptococcus, which revolutionized modern surgery and "robbed maternity of its chief dangers."[4] The bacillus of diphtheria and typhoid were also discovered in 1884.

All of these scientific discoveries — most of which originated in Europe — were utilized by public health officials in the United States to eradicate and inoculate against various diseases. The American Public Health Association (APHA) was formed in 1872 as a trade association for public health professionals and a clearinghouse of medical information. The *Journal of the American Public Health Association* began publication in 1895. Its early contents reveal that cholera and yellow fever were still raging virtually out of control in dozens of cities at the turn of the century. "Year after year we find pages devoted to the discussion of yellow fever" and early issues of the *Journal* contained titles like "The Germ Theory of Disease" and "Sewer Gas as a Cause of Scarlet Fever," notes Mazyck Ravenel, in his book *A Half Century of Public Health.*[5] Yellow fever, a scourge of the South ever since it was introduced into the United States in 1693, was not brought under control until 1900, the year in which the germ that causes the disease was discovered and a treatment applied.

The APHA's journal was renamed the *American Journal of Public Health* in 1912, a name that it still retains. In its early decades the focus of the association, as reflected in the titles of articles published in its journals, was the standardization of public health practices and methods throughout the nation. Early articles were written on "standard methods" for the examination of water and sewage, bacteriological examination of milk, examination of air, pasteurization of milk, model health codes for cities, and for public health training, among other topics.[6]

### Early Progress

The public health interventions of the late nineteenth and early twentieth century, which finally brought under control many communicable diseases such as cholera and yellow fever, resulted in a substantial reduction in mortality rates in America. In 1865, on the eve of the creation of the public health profession, the average annual death rate was about 25 per 1,000 population. By 1900 it had declined to 19 and by 1920 the rate had fallen to 14 per 1,000 population.[7]

Some of the declines in mortality rates for specific diseases were dramatic. For example, in Massachusetts the frequency of death from typhoid fever declined from a rate of 71.5 per 100,000 population in 1869 to 5.0 per 100,000 by 1920. Mortality from diphtheria among children was 65 per 10,000 for those under 15 years of age in 1879, but fell to 5 per 10,000 by 1920. The tuberculosis death rate in Massachusetts declined from more than 40 per 10,000 population in 1870 to 15 by 1918.

In Philadelphia from 1870 to 1920, death rates per 100,000 fell from 320 to 151 for tuberculosis; from 132 to 0 for smallpox; from 64 to 5 for typhoid fever; from 15 to 0 for dysentery; and from 7 to 0 for malaria. Such declines were "practically universal" throughout the country.[8]

Reviewing the first half-century's progress in public health, insurance industry statistician Frederick L. Hoffman concluded that "most of the important diseases which are looked upon as preventable or post-ponable have been reduced.... The diseases which are considered the efficiency test in health administration clearly emphasize that excellent and far-reaching results have followed initiative and energy in public health administration."[9]

Not all of the decline can be attributed to public health initiatives, however; increased economic prosperity is also very important. In fact, prosperity is arguably the *most* important determinant of improvements in the public's health; it enables us to improve our diet, housing, education, and medical care, among other things, that are so important to health. Wealthier is healthier.

## Major Public Health Developments

Many of the public health protections that we take for granted today — quarantines, sanitation, and so on — were revolutionary at the turn of the century and were of very high marginal (and total) value, to use economic terminology. That is, they provided a very big bang for the public health buck.

Until 1878 state and local governments were responsible for quarantining disease victims or ships docked in their harbors. In that year Congress first appropriated funds for "investigating the origin and causes of epidemic diseases, especially yellow fever and cholera, and the best method of preventing their introduction and spread," and assigned medical officers of the Public Health Service (then known as the Marine Hospital Service) to foreign consulates to supervise the enforcement of sanitary measures applicable to ships leaving for ports of the United States.[10] The federal government eventually took over all quarantine functions from state and local governments. As of 1921 the federal government administered "every [quarantine] station in the United States and in the Hawaiian Islands, the Philippines, Porto Rico [*sic*], and the Virgin Islands."[11]

In 1920 the quarantinable diseases found on ships were cholera, typhus, plague, smallpox, leprosy, and anthrax; other infectious diseases, such as measles, whooping cough, scarlet fever, and typhoid, were given no special quarantine treatment. Because of this quarantine system, outbreaks of disease were stopped in their tracks at a time — the turn of the century — when there was massive immigration from Europe and even Mexico, where disease was often more pervasive than in the United States. In one typical year (1921):

at national quarantine stations there were inspected approximately 2,000,000 passengers and crew. Twenty thousand vessels were inspected, and 5,000 were fumigated or disinfected. Three thousand nine hundred eighty-six vessels arrived from infected ports, of which number approximately 47 had infection aboard. Somewhat less than 50,000 passengers and crew were detained and disinfected; 4,800 were either vaccinated or subjected to bacteriological examination.[12]

The quarantine functions of government were nationalized in 1878, but state and local government health departments retained significant roles in public health. In 1921 the American Public Health Association listed the following items as typical areas of supervision for municipal health departments: housing, plumbing nuisances, vital statistics, contagious diseases, vaccination, infant hygiene, school inspection, industrial hygiene, health centers, public health nursing, food and drug regulation, milk regulation, garbage collection, health education, and publicity.[13]

Nuisance regulation involved eliminating filth caused by such things as pig pens, cesspools, privy vaults, and manure piles, all of which (one hopes!) no longer exist in the nation's cities. Milk regulation required pasteurization, and school inspection employed thousands of nurses in public schools to check school children for various diseases. The education and publicity functions involve educating the public in how to minimize the likelihood of contracting disease and what to do about it if one does.

In 1900 barely a million Americans lived in cities where the water supply was filtered. Shortly thereafter, another major public health improvement was the development and spread of municipal water filtration — to extract algae, certain minerals, pollution, and other substances — and disinfection of water supplies with chlorine. Water purification was especially effective in all but eliminating typhoid fever.

Other turn-of-the-century public health achievements included improved sewage and solid waste removal and treatment procedures in cities, pollution control, and the promotion of private voluntary agencies devoted to child nutrition and overall health. For example, the Child Health Organization of America, founded in 1918, crusaded for modest but effective health measures such as a scale in every school, time allotted in each school day for teaching health, hot school lunches, teacher training in health, and "every child's weight to be taken and the record sent home every month."[14] The Girl Scouts (incorporated in 1915), Boy Scouts, Camp Fire Girls, and the Little Mothers' Leagues were other national organizations devoted to teaching children the principles of hygiene.

As the nation became more industrialized "industrial hygiene" became a major concern of public health professionals. Close attention was paid to the economic costs of sickness and temporary disability due to on-the-job injuries. In 1917, a national commission estimated that 875,000 people were disabled for four weeks or more by industrial accidents. Seventy-five percent of the accidents, the commission concluded, were preventable.[15] A greater degree of individual responsibility for one's physical fitness, health, and hygiene was stressed, because it was widely recognized that the main cause of industrial accidents then, as now, was human error or carelessness.

Early twentieth-century public health departments were dominated by physicians who, though they supported some kinds of government intervention, such as quarantines, inoculations, and health education, were wary of any trends toward the incremental governmental takeover of the private practice of medicine. For example, in 1921 the American Medical Association opposed (unsuccessfully) federal legislation that funded child health programs by state departments of health. "The AMA saw this as the opening wedge for the provision of all medical care by government" and, while it saw *some* role for public health interventions, it "vigorously opposed proposals for compulsory National Health Insurance."[16]

Table 2.1 shows that for its first fifty years the elected leaders of the APHA were exclusively physicians or medical researchers whose careers were devoted to public health research, education, and treatment of patients. They were widely published in medical journals and received many awards for their scientific achievements.

By contrast, as will be seen in later chapters, many of today's public health leaders are much more likely to be political activists whose interests and training are in social welfare policy rather than the natural sciences and the study of medicine, per se.

## Public Health Department Functions in Contemporary America

A 1990 survey of local government health departments revealed that the functions reported by the nation's 3,000 or so local health departments still focus on disease research, control, immunization, and public education (table 2.2).

A different survey by the American Public Health Association found that other health departments provide such additional services as dental health services (fluoridation, dental health education in schools),

TABLE 2.1

APHA Presidents, 1872-1922

| President/Year Elected | Area of Specialization |
| --- | --- |
| Stephen Smith (1872) | Surgery |
| Joseph Toner (1875) | Medical biographer/writer |
| John Henry Rauch (1877) | Medical botany, sanitary science |
| Elisha Harris (1877) | Sanitation, hygiene, medical statistics |
| James Cabell (1878) | Anatomy, physiology, surgery |
| John S. Billings (1879) | Medical statistics |
| Robert Kedzie (1881) | Chemistry and sanitary science |
| Ezra Hunt (1882) | Anatomy |
| Albert Gihon (1883) | Hygiene |
| George Sternberg (1885) | Bacteriology |
| Emanuel Lachapelle (1893) | Sanitarian |
| William Bailey (1894) | Sanitarian |
| Eduardo Liceaga (1895) | Hygiene/Surgery |
| Henry Horlbeck (1896) | Surgery |
| Benjamin Lee (1900) | Orthopedic Surgery |
| Henry Holton (1901) | Surgery |
| Walter Wyman (1902) | Surgery/Quarantine procedures |
| Carlos Finlay (1903) | Bacteriology |
| Frank Wesbrook (1905) | Pathology and Bacteriology |
| Franklin Robinson (1905) | Chemistry and public health |
| Domingo Orvananos (1906) | Internal medicine |
| William Sedgwick (1914) | Bacteriology |

*Source*: Mazyck P. Ravenel, ed. *A Half Century of Public Health* (New York: Arno Press, 1970), pp. 30-55.

substance abuse services, education about accident protection, inspection of beaches and recreational areas, radiation protection, sanitation in schools, prisons and hospitals, emergency medical services, medical care for prison inmates, and mental health diagnosis and treatment.[17] The direct provision of medical care by government health departments primarily serves low-income Americans, but many of the services listed above obviously affect everyone regardless of income.

State health departments also exist in each state, with many of their functions overlapping those of the local health departments. One sur-

TABLE 2.2

**Functions of Local Public Health Departments**

| | |
|---|---|
| Reportable disease collection and analysis | Communicable disease epidemiology |
| Public health policy priority setting | Public health planning |
| Health code development/enforcement | Inspection activity |
| Licensing | Health education |
| Hazardous waste management | Solid waste management |
| Water pollution monitoring and control | Insect and animal control |
| Water supply safety | Sewage disposal systems |
| Laboratory services | Handicapped children's assistance |
| Home health care | AIDS testing and counseling |
| Prenatal care | Family planning |
| Prevention of chronic diseases | Control of sexually transmitted |
| Administering federal Women, Infants, | diseases |
| and Children (WIC) programs | Child health |
| Immunization programs | |

*Source*: *1990 National Profile of Local Health Departments*, cited in George E. and Terry W. Pickett, *Opportunities in Public Health Careers* (Lincolnwood, Ill.: NTC Publishing Group, 1995), p. 30.

vey found the following functions performed by state health departments (table 2.3).

Like the local health department functions, many of these are said to possess "public goods" features, such as the administration of quarantines, pollution control, and communicable disease control. Other functions are primarily income redistribution programs that provide free in-kind services to lower-income citizens. Some other services are purely private services that are also provided by for-profit businesses — refuse disposal, alcohol and addiction services, ambulance service, home health care, nursing, extermination services, and emergency medical services. Thus, to some extent, state and local governments have "crowded out" or displaced private-sector businesses that provide, or could provide, many of the same services.[18] Taxpayer subsidies and the frequent exemption from regulations that burden for-profit businesses give governments an unfair advantage over for-profit firms. Sometimes no competition at all is permitted; the governments providing the services enjoy legal monopolies established by local legislation.

Sometimes, the government provision of "public health services" may have less to do with public health than the protection of a certain dominant industry or specialty. Consider the provision of occupational licensing. An especially egregious example of this phenomenon occurred recently in Maryland.

TABLE 2.3

### Functions of State Health Departments

| | |
|---|---|
| Communicable disease control | Vital statistics |
| Promulgation of rules and regulations | Venereal disease control |
| Quarantines | Tuberculosis control |
| Water pollution control | Facilities inspection |
| Facilities licensure | Laboratory services |
| Refuse disposal | Air pollution control |
| Abating of nuisances/filth | Health education |
| Radiological health | Food inspection |
| Mental health | Prevention of blindness |
| Maternal and child health | Immunizations |
| Occupational health | Indigent care |
| Chronic disease control | Crippled children services |
| Milk inspection | Housing inspection |
| Alcohol and addiction control services | Dental health |
| Establishment of local hospitals | Rabies control |
| Ambulance services | School health |
| Home health care | Nursing care |
| Family planning | Extermination services |
| Nutrition programs | Emergency medical services |

Source: Marshall and Norma Raffel, *The U.S. Health System: Origins and Functions* (New York: Wiley, 1989), p. 268.

On Maryland's eastern shore a small number of low-income, elderly women, most of whom are widows, earn their income by picking the meat out of crabs caught by local fishermen and selling the meat to restaurants to prepare Maryland's famous crab cakes. At the insistence of larger, commercial seafood companies the Maryland Health Department decided to regulate the women by requiring that they purchase "proper" equipment, including stainless steel tables, which would cost them approximately $50,000 each, according to local news reports.

No one claimed that there was a public health threat; the state simply decided to regulate the women out of business. The beneficiaries were the corporate interests who apparently felt threatened by competition from the women. The losers would be the women themselves, as well as the restaurants' customers who would pay somewhat higher prices for crabmeat because of the diminished competition.

This is just one small example, but the creation of barriers to occupational entry under the guise of health regulation is so pervasive that civil rights attorney Clint Bolick has written a book about it with the ominous title, *Grassroots Tyranny*.[19]

## The Federal Role in Public Health

In the U.S. House of Representatives there are twenty committees and thirty-three subcommittees that play a role in public health matters. In the Senate there are seventeen committees and twenty-three subcommittees concerned with health affairs. Thus, virtually every member of Congress is on some committee related to public health. Some commentators believe this is an efficient arrangement since it allows full committees to delegate much of the work. But scholars have also pointed out that the proliferation of subcommittees is more likely the result of the desire by members of Congress to help ensure their own reelection by being able to target federal money for myriad purposes, including public health. Members of Congress want to be on a health-related committee because the federal government dispenses billions of dollars annually for hundreds of individual public health programs administered at the state and local levels of government.

Moreover, the disbursement of funds guarantees that "local" public health policy is effectively controlled by the federal government, for federal funds always come with strings attached that restrict the use of the money. Federal programs tend to impose "one-size-fits-all" policies that may be appropriate in some areas but totally inappropriate in others. For example, one would think that an appropriate clean air policy for Los Angeles, California, would be radically different than one for Bozeman, Montana, yet the Environmental Protection Agency imposes uniform auto emissions and other policies for all regions of the country. The federal role in public health has become pervasive, as indicated by the amount of official study devoted to it; the General Accounting Office conducts studies of various health issues; the Congressional Budget Office evaluates the fiscal impact of health policies. The Department of Health and Human Services, arguably the largest government bureaucracy in the world, intervenes in almost every aspect of human health — and many areas that are only remotely related to it.

The Public Health Service is the one agency within HHS that is most directly related to public health. Its stated objectives are: preventing and controlling disease, identifying health hazards, promoting healthy lifestyles, assisting in the delivery of health care services, administering block grants to the states for health services, "ensuring" that drugs and medical devices are safe and effective, protecting the public from unsafe foods and "unnecessary exposure" to "man-made radiation," conducting and supporting biomedical research, and working with other nations on "global health problems."[20]

Such a far-reaching, self-defined job description gives the Public Health Service an almost unlimited capacity for growth. If it carried out all of its self-professed objectives, it would have to intervene in almost all aspects of our daily lives.

The National Institutes of Health (NIH) is the medical research arm of the Public Health Service. Its research moneys are distributed to its twelve research units: the National Cancer Institute, National Institute on Aging, National Institute of Child Health and Human Development, National Institute of General Medical Sciences, National Heart, Lung and Blood Institute, National Institute of Allergy and Infectious Diseases, National Institute of Dental Research, National Institute of Neurological and Communicative Disorders and Stroke, National Institute of Arthritis and Musculoskeletal and Skin Diseases, National Institute of Diabetes and Digestive and Kidney Diseases, National Institute of Environmental Health Sciences, National Eye Institute, and the National Center for Nursing Research.[21]

Other federal public health bureaucracies include the Alcohol, Drug Abuse, and Mental Health Administration, the Food and Drug Administration, Centers for Disease Control, National Center for Health Statistics, Health Resources and Services Administration, Health Care Financing Administration, Occupational Safety and Health Administration, Environmental Protection Agency, and parts of the Federal Trade Commission.

This federal intervention in the name of "public health" began in the 1930s with the increased funding of state and local public health functions through the Social Security Act. This activity maybe constitutionally questionable, however.

One textbook on public health states that "the Constitution ... grants to Congress the power to regulate foreign and interstate commerce. This justifies much of the federal activity regarding regulation of foods, drugs, product and occupational safety, and some environmental health activities, because they move in, or affect, interstate or foreign commerce."[22] This is a perversion of the Commerce Clause. The clause was intended to *limit* governmental power and to serve as a negative check on government intervention, not to provide carte blanche powers to the federal bureaucracy.

The original purpose of the Commerce Clause was to allow the federal government to strike down protectionist tariffs imposed by individual states that impeded interstate commerce. Early rulings also prohibited states from granting monopoly rights to steamship companies. As economic historians Terry Anderson and P.J. Hill observed, until the 1870s "the commerce clause was a negative check on the state interference with interstate commerce rather than a positive guide for federal intervention.... Before the Civil War, the sole use of the commerce clause by the Supreme Court was to negate state statutes."[23]

An extreme example of how the Commerce Clause has been reinterpreted in the name of "public health" is illustrated in a dissent to the 1995 decision of the U.S. Supreme Court (*Lopez vs. U.S.*), which ruled a federal gun control law to be unconstitutional. Congress had passed a law restricting possession of firearms within a certain distance from school buildings. The court ruled that the federal government had no authority in the matter, that such laws were the domain of local governments. In his dissent, Justice Stephen Breyer argued that since the law affected education and since education in turn affects labor productivity, which in turn affects interstate commerce, the federal government should have a right to regulate all aspects of local education. Such is the thinking that has brought us a long way from Jefferson's admonition that government should be "bound by the chains of the Constitution."

"It is the general welfare clause that justifies support for medical research, Medicare, Medicaid, health employee training, and so on," says a typical public health text.[24] But this, too, is a stretch. Many government programs benefit only small segments of the population, not the *general* public. Moreover, the general welfare clause was originally designed to assure *uniform taxation* to finance genuine public goods. In reality, virtually all federal taxation is discriminatory — different rates are paid by different citizens — and it finances special benefits to narrowly defined groups. Indeed, contemporary proponents of the privatization of Medicare consider the program to be a "public bad," not a public good. As University of Chicago legal scholar Richard Epstein has concluded, "the developments under the commerce clause and the general welfare clause show once again how easily the Supreme Court can convert a charter of limited government into one of plenary legislative power."[25]

## Public Health and Public Policy

The American Public Health Association publishes a compendium of the association's public policy statements from 1948 to the present which provides an interesting look into how the association's priorities have shifted in the past half century.[26] (This shifting emphasis will be the focus of the next several chapters). The policy statements are in the form of resolutions or position papers worked out by various committees of the association before being considered by a joint policy committee, which includes members of an "action board" that is involved in "social and political action." A governing council decides by vote which proposals are accepted and become official APHA policy.

During the late 1940s and 1950s the policy proposals of the APHA were largely in keeping with the traditional public health focus of providing public goods through controlling communicable disease, public education, etc. In the late 1940s the association's resolutions were devoted to such issues as encouraging more research on child development, marriage, and occupational safety, along with promoting health education in schools, the education of nurses, rehabilitating the disabled, promoting the fluoridation of public water supplies, and better collection of statistics on nutrition, marriage and divorce, and industrial mortality rates.[27]

One 1949 resolution in particular stands out, however, because it is so out of character with *today's* public health movement. Resolution 4901 states that "present federal and state taxes on oleomargarine seriously raise the retail price of this commodity, thus violating the principle that government should facilitate rather than hinder the provision of a satisfactory diet for all the people." Thus, the association "condemns specific taxes on oleomargarine ... and respectfully petitions the Congress and the various state legislatures to repeal these taxes."[28]

As will be seen in later chapters, the public health movement in America has become almost as much of a lobbyist for an enlarged welfare state as a vehicle for promoting public health. A call for cutting taxes — any taxes — would today be unlikely. Back in 1949 when the main "constituents" of public health professionals were the residents of the cities and states from which they derived most of their funding, they were obviously concerned about such matters as how "sin taxes" on oleomargarine pinched the family budget. But now that so much funding of public health comes from Washington, calling for reductions in federal excise taxes would be considered biting the hand that feeds you — even if it would help the public, especially low-income families. Indeed, public health professionals are vigorous lobbyists for higher excise taxes on many items, because the revenues derived from the taxes are sometimes earmarked as supplements to public health budgets.

Another 1950 resolution that is noteworthy is Resolution 5013, announcing that the association "does not now advocate any one method of financing" medical care.[29] Beginning in the 1960s, however, the association embraced and actively promoted government control of medical care in the form of national health insurance, euphemistically referred to today as a "single-payer system."

# 3

# Birth of the "New Public Health"

*"Socialism has come to mean chiefly the extensive
redistribution of incomes through taxation and the
institutions of the welfare state."*

—*Friedrich Hayek*, The Road to Serfdom

The APHA's public policy statements reveal that throughout the 1950s the public health establishment focused primarily on health-related "public goods" provision — its traditional function. It promoted such policies as the fluoridation of public water supplies, research on occupational and industrial mortality, more stringent sanitation standards, research and education on periodontal disease, the eradication of malaria, accident prevention education, and education efforts regarding the health hazards of "excessive cigarette smoking."[1]

This last item alone gives an indication of the change that has occurred in public health policy. In the 1950s the thinking was that "excessive smoking," like excessive eating or drinking, involved health risks, and that public health professionals should inform the public — especially children — of these risks. It was hoped that citizens would refrain from smoking, given this information, but there was no effort to ban smoking.

By contrast, today's public health movement is much more prohibitionist. Educating the public is not enough. Laws must be passed that will lead to a "smoke-free society"— one of the favorite catch phrases of the modern anti-smoking movement.

Another striking policy change over the past several decades has to do with the APHA's stance on the licensing of doctors. In the early 1990s the APHA endorsed and promoted the failed Clinton administration plan to nationalize the medical care sector, complete with governmental edicts to *reduce* the supposedly "excessive" number of medical specialists. Although the plan was abandoned by the administration in 1994, some of it has been adopted piecemeal since then. In late 1996, for instance, the administration announced that it was going to pay teaching hospitals in New York for *not* training physicians, similar to the decades-old policy of paying farmers for not growing crops or raising livestock. These agricultural policies have long been recognized by economists as cartel price-fixing schemes, which are fundamentally anti-consumer because they force up the price of food and otherwise distort supply and demand in agricultural markets, all the while costing taxpayers billions of dollars.[2]

By contrast, consider a 1960 resolution by the APHA, which was more in keeping with promoting the general interests of the public and holding down the costs of medical care: "Whereas the present acute national shortage of well-trained physicians is expected to persist and cannot be overcome for at least one or two decades," the resolution read, and "Whereas the medical licensure laws of some states are unduly restrictive...," the APHA called for less restrictive licensing laws that would not create such severe barriers to entry into the medical profession. The association's objective was "to minimize the barriers to licensure of qualified physicians in the several states."[3]

An equally stark change of opinion appears in the area of environmental policy. Today, the public health association has become closely aligned with the political agenda of the extremist environmental movement — even though certain environmental polices may adversely affect the public's health. Yet, back in 1963, the association took a much more balanced and scientific perspective on environmental matters than prevails today. For example, a resolution issued in that year called for "Enhancement of public awareness of the *benefits and hazards* of pesticides" (emphasis added).[4] Such language is a refreshing reminder that it is possible to discuss cost-benefit issues rationally rather than just blindly opposing the use of pesticides and ignoring or downplaying their role in controlling insects and disease and in assisting agriculture, while improving public health.

## Bureaucratic Incentives and the Federalization of Public Health

Having solved a number of genuine "public goods" problems —primarily the virtual eradication of many communicable diseases — the public health establishment faced a dilemma: Does solving the problems they were established to solve mean that there is no longer a need for such a large "establishment"? And if not, shouldn't tax dollars be diverted to more productive uses?

Like most bureaucracies, the public health establishment did not decide to "downsize" once its major mission was completed. Instead it reinvented and broadened its purpose, seeking additional federal funds to finance its growing agenda. This led to two fundamental changes. First, there was a movement away from activities that could be construed as the provision of public goods. Second, with a larger and larger portion of state and local public health budgets being financed by the federal government, federal priorities became increasingly important, sometimes to the detriment of local public health problems. As noted previously, Washington policymakers tend to impose "one-size-fits-all" programs on state and local governments. As a result, this federalization of public health has in many ways rendered state and local public health departments less effective in dealing with traditional public health problems.

Beginning in the early 1950s, when federal grants to state and local governments were initiated, the APHA championed federal funding for state and local public health programs, seemingly oblivious to the inevitable federal control that accompanies federal financing. The association issued a resolution in 1953 reminding everyone that it "has consistently favored the development of local health services as a requisite to safeguarding the health of the Nation," but then resolved to press Congress for more federal tax dollars in support of local public health.

By the mid 1960s, the APHA would completely abandon many of its earlier positions. Consider its opinion that excise taxes on food items were deleterious to a "satisfactory diet" and public health, held throughout the 1950s (as noted in chapter 2). In 1965 the association declared that the "development of all possible tax sources at the state level is a necessity..." and advocated "improved tax sharing" by the federal government.[5] From that point on the public health establishment became one of many lobbyists for tax increases "from all possible tax sources," presumably including food, clothing, shelter, medicine, and pharmaceuticals. Its demands for tax dollars began to supersede its concern for promoting public health.

## Public Health's Point of Demarcation

As of 1963 the public health establishment still defined the "functions of the local health department" as "promotion of personal and community health; maintenance of a healthful environment; and an aggressive attack on disease and disability."[6] But during the 1960s it slowly began to change its focus from public health, per se, to social policy. Seriously concerned over its future financial stability, the establishment attached itself to the financial gravy train of the newly initiated "Great Society" welfare state programs of the Johnson administration. The "new public health" placed a premium on those with lobbying and public relations skills and who were more concerned with "social policy" than with such "mundane" problems as local mosquito abatement, inoculation against disease, and so on. No longer were the most prominent and influential public health professionals surgeons, sanitarians, hygienists, physiologists, chemists, bacteriologists, or pathologists.

The point of demarcation from traditional public health pursuits seems to have occurred in 1968 when the American Public Health Association enthusiastically endorsed the federal government's "Kerner Report" on the "root causes" of poverty, praising the report as one of "the most rational proposals for social health yet devised." The APHA declared that "We, as an Association, accept as our own the principles of the Kerner Report."[7]

Note the use of the word "social." A healthy "society" was now the apparent focus of the public health establishment. This simple change of language reflected a broadening of public health's self-defined mission to include such "health" issues as poverty, racism, and housing policy.

The Kerner Report advocated a number of welfare state policies that were adopted and funded with trillions of federal tax dollars over the past thirty years (about $7 trillion has been spent on welfare programs since 1967). These programs have not succeeded (as discussed below), but the APHA still vigorously supports their expansion and opposes most proposals for fundamental reform of the failed programs.

The Kerner Report recommended "creating" one million government jobs in just three years; a "national system of income supplementation ... for all Americans"; a massive increase in welfare payments to unwed mothers; the building of six million government housing units over five years; an expanded "rent supplement program" for those living in government housing projects; a massive expansion of the Department of Health, Education, and Welfare (now the Department of Health and Human Services) in order to enforce affirmative action programs more effectively; the adoption of racial hiring quotas as prerequisites for federal construction contracts (so-called "equal opportunity for employment by federal contractors"); and school busing ostensibly to achieve school integration.

In less than a century the public health profession had evolved from one concerned primarily with sanitation, disease, hygiene, clean air and water, and other matters directly related to improving the healthiness of everyday living, to lobbyists and advocates for an enlarged welfare state. The route to "public health" was transformed from efforts to control disease to efforts to *affect* living standards by controlling behavior and income. This involved direct government intervention through welfare programs.

The word socialism is not too strong a term to describe the APHA's policy focus. Using the tax system to redistribute income — public health's new, top priority as of 1968 — may be thought of as the American version of socialism. As Nobel laureate Friedrich Hayek explained in the 1976 preface to his international classic, *The Road to Serfdom*, from the initial printing of the book in 1944 to 1976 "terminology has changed.... At the time I wrote, socialism meant unambiguously the nationalization of the means of production and the central economic planning which this made possible and necessary." But today "socialism has come to mean chiefly the extensive redistribution of incomes through taxation and the institutions of the welfare state."[8]

Thus, since 1968 a top priority — if not *the* top priority — of the public health establishment has been to promote the idea that more government control and intervention is the surest route to sounder health. This proposition is dubious at best. World events have clearly revealed that the many variants of socialism have one thing in common: They create numerous and serious economic and social problems. Beyond some minimal level (protection of private property, enforcement of contracts, national defense, a judicial system, basic infrastructure, including public health infrastructure), government intervention impedes economic growth and, therefore, contributes to poverty. And more poverty means a *less* healthy society — precisely the opposite of public health.

Equating "public health" with a more socialist society is still a top priority of the American Public Health Association and of many public health professionals. As Sally Satel, a physician, wrote in the *Wall Street Journal*, in the field of public health "activist researchers — some of whom aren't doctors or epidemiologists but sociologists or cultural anthropologists — are moving the field in a pernicious direction."[9]

Dr. Satel attended the 1996 annual convention of the APHA where the keynote speaker was not a physician or medical researcher, but AFL-CIO president John Sweeney, who asked the attendees to "help us rejuvenate the labor movement." The conference was apparently a real eye opener for the doctor, who was surprised to discover that the theme of the conference had little to do with science, medicine, or even traditional public health issues. Indeed, the official theme was "Empowering the Disadvantaged: Social Justice in Public Health." Little has changed since 1968: Public health is still defined by the activist leaders of the movement as more government regulation and intervention.

Among the "prescriptions" for improving public health that were discussed at the conference were "radical redistribution of wealth" because "living in an unjust society damages physical health."[10] Illness is supposedly caused by a "power imbalance" that is supposedly "inherent in a capitalist society" which is why the free market must be "counteracted" with "social programs."

As a practicing physician, Dr. Satel was appalled at the conference's predominant "world view that regards the patient as a passive victim of malign social forces." Some of the greatest successes in public health, she wrote, "have involved efforts to change personal behavior by educating the public about the risks of such activities as smoking, unhealthy eating and unprotected sex.... More than half of all premature deaths are attributable to risky personal behavior."[11]

The political activists who promote this world view were not fazed by Dr. Satel's criticism. They defended their political activism in letters-to-the-editor by reiterating their convictions that "social conditions" can be a major cause of public health problems. The *Journal* published three such letters under the heading, "Social Justice Equals Public Health," an accurate definition of the philosophy of "the new public health."

In a telephone conversation with one of the authors, Dr. Satel stated that she did not disagree at all with the proposition that such "social conditions" as poverty contributed to health problems. The problem with the public health establishment is that it believes socialism to be the "cure" for these problems, contrary to voluminous evidence in the economics literature — not to mention the world's experiences over the past several decades.

Among the other prominent new positions taken by the APHA during the 1960s is the 1968 declaration that "the factors in our social system which reduce and perpetuate poverty" are "substandard and insufficient education, housing, health services, and welfare services."[12] And the way to provide these things is through government, not the private enterprise system. Thus, what is needed is a vast expansion of the nation's "inadequate, inequitable, and inefficient welfare system."[13]

The APHA also adopted the questionable view that individuals are not responsible for their own health. Accepting the idea that individuals are ultimately responsible for their own well-being — once a central tenet of the public health movement — leads one naturally to the conclusion that the most effective efforts of public health professionals are educational — research and education provided to citizens on how they can lead healthier lives.

This philosophy was officially dropped in 1968 when the APHA declared that "Government holds ultimate accountability for the nation's health."[14] This is more in keeping with the point of view that "social forces" tend to "victimize" hapless citizens, harming their health. In accordance with this perspective, "activists" work to "save" defenseless citizens from evil social forces. Thus, "social programs" are needed to cure disease, not medical research, education, and patient care.

The APHA also climbed aboard the zero-population-growth bandwagon during the 1960s and 1970s by openly endorsing abortion on demand and taxpayer-financed "sterilization for men and women."[15] Government control of medical care is perhaps the one overriding policy objective of the APHA: "A national program for universal, comprehensive, personal health services is required as a basic guarantee of equal opportunity for good health."[16] Such a program would declare government-funded health care to be a "social right" and would have government set prices for medical care (price controls). Nationalizing the health insurance industry also became a key objective.

In the early 1970s the APHA advocated central planning for the energy industry in the form of a "coherent and comprehensive energy policy" and also endorsed centrally planned land use because of fears of the "unknown health effects of open space." This seems especially odd in light of the fact that the public health profession was created to address problems caused by *not enough* open space, that is, urbanization.

The APHA also endorsed during the 1970s most of the most extreme positions of the political environmental movement, including a harsh condemnation of the automobile (not too different from Vice President Al Gore's call for elimination of the internal combustion engine in his book, *Earth in the Balance*). In 1973 the association warned ominously that "the automobile presents an immediate health and safety hazard through death and maiming in highway accidents and a longer range health danger through air and noise pollution."[17] Individual drivers or polluters are not to be held responsible, according to the APHA, but the automobile, per se. Such thinking has led the political environmental movement in the direction of a regulatory attack on the automobile which has driven up the cost of the average car while providing few health benefits. The ultimate objective seems to be tight restrictions on the use of automobiles, not necessarily to improve public health.

### Economic Ignorance Is Hazardous to Public Health

As Dr. Satel explained, many of the researchers and "activists" in today's public health movement are not physicians or medical researchers, but are often sociologists, cultural anthropologists, and other non-medical professionals. There is also an almost complete absence of economic knowledge in the movement, as evidenced by its promotion of welfare schemes.

For example, the APHA since 1968 has supported government "jobs programs" to combat unemployment. But the creation of government jobs has never been able to reduce unemployment because of the economic law of opportunity cost, a lesson that is taught to every college student (and many high school students) during the first weeks of principles of economics. Specifically, because government jobs must be financed either by taxing, government borrowing, or governmental money creation via the Federal Reserve, resources are necessarily diverted from the private sector of the economy to pay for the jobs in the public sector. Taxes take money out of citizen's pockets; government borrowing pushes up interest rates and reallocates financial capital to government-preferred uses, crowding out private borrowing for home and appliance purchases, business creation and expansion, and myriad other uses; and money creation creates inflation, which reduces the value of all privately held wealth. In other words, government "jobs programs" can only *reallocate* the kinds of jobs that exist — more government jobs and fewer private-sector jobs — but they cannot "create" jobs. Only private-sector entrepreneurs can create jobs.

Moreover, government "jobs programs" tend to destroy jobs because they typically cost considerably more than the amount of money spent on salaries because of the cost of bureaucratic overhead. Past government jobs programs have spent well over $100,000 for each $15,000-per-year job "created." That is why even the Democratic-controlled

Congress voted to kill the totally ineffective CETA (Comprehensive Employment and Training Act) program in the late 1970s.

The APHA also seems unaware of the ineffectiveness of welfare in reducing poverty and to its counterproductive effects on work incentives, family stability, and other social problems. Both major political parties have recognized that the American welfare programs has largely failed, which is why the Republican-controlled Congress and the Clinton White House agreed in 1996 to reform the system and even to phase out one of the largest welfare programs, AFDC (Aid to Families With Dependent Children). But the APHA continues to criticize such reforms and advocates an even larger welfare state. In short, the "activists" in the public health movement are unreconstructed 1960s-era leftists who use "health" to promote their political agenda of income redistribution through the tax system and an enlarged welfare state.

The effects of welfare on work incentives in the United States have been pernicious. Harvard sociologist William Julius Wilson has recently written about the phenomenon of the virtually complete absence of adults who work for a living in many inner-city, predominantly black, neighborhoods. What Professor Wilson fails to recognize or acknowledge, however, is that the most important reason why work has "disappeared" from some American neighborhoods is that welfare payments in many areas of the country literally make it uneconomical to choose to work.

Economist Stephen Moore of the Cato Institute, in Washington, D.C., recently calculated the wages one would have to earn in each state in order to enjoy the same standard of living that one could enjoy by receiving benefits from the seven most popular welfare programs. On average, an American welfare recipient would have to earn about $10 an hour and as much as $18 an hour (in Hawaii) in order to "break even," because as one's earned income increases welfare benefits decline. Since very few welfare recipients can earn $10 an hour, and since even if they could, it would hardly seem worth the bother if one could do just as well by not working and remaining on welfare, the American welfare system has trapped millions of people on welfare by undermining the financial incentives to work.

The "activists" in the public health movement, who for several decades have lobbied for higher and higher levels of welfare payments, have contributed to this serious problem. This is not the place to present a comprehensive summary of the effects of the American welfare state. But it is noteworthy that the ill effects of the welfare system are not only economic but also psychological. As political scientist Charles Murray has written,

> It is essential to the pursuit of happiness that one earn one's life. The threshold condition of self-respect is that one feel, not in one's public protestations but in one's heart, that he is a net contributor to the world.... An acceptable social policy is one that validates the individual's responsibility for the consequences of his behavior....A social policy that induces people to believe that they are not responsible for their lives is one that inhibits the pursuit of happiness and is to that extent immoral.[18]

As noted above, the basic premise of "the new public health" is that people are not, in fact, responsible for their own lives but are buffeted about by often malign "social forces" such as capitalism.

For the past thirty years the APHA has also politically supported government housing, another failure. The lack of individual property rights dooms all government housing projects, inevitably, to become dilapidated slums. People simply do not take as good care of "public" property as they do their own. In the absence of property rights housing rapidly deteriorates, making the "housing problem" even worse. The public health establishment's support for "decent housing" is a quixotic quest if by "decent housing" it means building more government housing projects.

In response to the *Wall Street Journal* article by Dr. Sally Satel, Professor Nancy Krieger of the Harvard School of Public Health's department of health and social behavior wrote a letter to the *Journal* informing Dr. Satel and others that "efforts to improve health behaviors are most successful among those who can afford to live well," and argued that "public welfare must be placed before corporate welfare and social equality before unrestricted freedom of the economic market."[19] Three other letters by Barry Levy, president of the APHA, Vincent Iacopino of Physicians for Human Rights, and Ronald David of the Kennedy School of Government at Harvard echoed Professor Kreiger's remarks.

Coming from the president of the APHA and faculty members at Harvard's Kennedy School of Government and its School of Public Health, it is reasonable to think of these remarks as fairly representative of the views of the leaders and activists of "the new public health." What they also represent is a view of the economic world whereby the welfare of "corporations" is necessarily at odds with the welfare of average citizens, and free markets are harmful to public health, whereas massive government income redistribution programs ("social equality") are helpful.

Overwhelming evidence that this view of the economic world is backwards is presented in three voluminous studies of economic freedom around the world by Freedom House, Canada's Fraser Institute, and the Heritage Foundation and *Wall Street Journal*.[20] The study by Freedom House, the New York-based human rights organization known for its annual surveys of the state of political freedom in the world, surveyed the degree of "economic freedom" in countries around the world. "In most nations privatization of state enterprises, the lifting of wage and price controls and the removal of other direct restraints on economic life have become the accepted wisdom," wrote the study's editor, Richard E. Messick.[21] Those countries that do the best job of deregulating their economies and enforcing the rule of law, which means "at a minimum ... creating an environment where force and fraud are suppressed, contracts enforced and property rights defined," experience the most vigorous economic growth.[22] "There is an extraordinary correlation between economic freedom, and growth and prosperity," said Mr. Messick.[23]

The Freedom House "Indicators of Economic Freedom" included freedom to hold property, earn a living, operate a business, invest one's earnings, engage in international trade, and participate in the market economy generally. The report found that twenty-seven "economically free" nations, with 17 percent of the world's population, account for 81 percent of the world's total output of goods and services. There are no inherent limits to the spread of economic freedom and prosperity, the study concluded, although many governments "refuse to extend their citizens these fundamental rights."[24] There is also a close link between economic and political freedom, according to Freedom House. Those countries that have achieved a relatively high degree of economic freedom also tend to have more political freedom as well.

The Fraser Institute study constructed an economic freedom index with seventeen components grouped into four broad areas: Money and Inflation, Government Regulation, Takings and Discriminatory Taxation, and Restrictions on International Exchange. The central elements of economic freedom, according to this study, are "personal choice, protection of private property, and freedom of exchange."[25]

The Fraser Institute study found that the fourteen countries that earned "grades" of "A" or "B" in its rankings achieved average annual economic growth per capita of 2.6 percent from 1985 to 1994; the twenty-seven countries graded as "F" experienced an average annual "growth" rate per capita of *minus* 1.6 percent for the 1985-1994 period. Furthermore, no country in the Fraser Institute study that maintained persistently high economic freedom ratings failed to achieve a high level of income and the countries with the largest increases in economic freedom during the period under study achieved impressive growth rates.

The Heritage Foundation/*Wall Street Journal* study was very similar to the Fraser Institute and Freedom House projects and concluded that "countries with the highest levels of economic freedom also have the highest living standards. Similarly, countries with the lowest levels of economic freedom also have the lowest living standards."[26] It also revealed an interesting (but discouraging) phenomenon: "Wealthy and economically free countries tend to reintroduce restrictions on economic freedom over time. As they become wealthy, countries begin adding welfare and other social programs that were not affordable when they were poorer ... the seeds of [economic] destruction can exist in the fruits of success."[27]

These findings have crucially important implications for public health and for the state of the public health profession. There is overwhelming evidence that freer economies, ones that allow government the role of enforcing "the rules of the game" but permit little interference in the market place and keep taxing and spending to relatively low levels, are the most prosperous. And economic prosperity, which can only be created by private sector entrepreneurs and workers, is conducive to both a higher degree of political freedom and the enhancement of public health. All of the social problems the public health establishment is so concerned about — poverty, adequate housing, hunger, and so on — are solved most efficiently by higher levels of economic growth. Because economic freedom is a prerequisite for economic growth, the public health establishment's advocacy of more government involvement in the economy is a hindrance to achieving greater prosperity and improving public health.

## Attacking the Profit Motive

The public health movement has long criticized the institutions of private property, private enterprise, and profit seeking in the health care field. There is self-interest at work here; after all, government-financed hospitals, nursing homes, and other health care institutions in the government and nonprofit sectors compete with proprietary, for-profit institutions. A critique of profit seeking by the American Public Health

Association is the same as, say, the American Automobile Manufacturers' Association criticizing Japanese automakers. Nevertheless, in 1975 the APHA declared that "health care, unlike most other services and commodities, is a life and death matter which is hazardous to leave to the pressures of the profit motive."[28] Consequently, the association urged the government to "monitor" carefully all aspects of proprietary health care provision and supported "a full scale study" of the effects of profit-making corporations in the health sector.

Because the APHA favors government control of medical care, the association has publicly stated that it is opposed to the expansion of private sector health providers (hospitals, nursing homes, etc.). The proliferation of private-sector health care providers, in the APHA's view, makes it more difficult to increase government's role in health care.

The public health establishment usually opposes any reform of health care that would move in the direction of greater reliance on competition, private enterprise, and consumer choice. The APHA even criticized the failed Clinton health plan in 1993 — which would have abolished the private health insurance industry and put the federal government in charge of most of the health care market — as being "too market oriented"!

There is evidence, however, that the public health establishment's views toward profit-seeking in the health care sector are as misguided as its views of economic freedom and economic growth in general are. A major study of for-profit health care institutions was published in the *Harvard Business Review* by Regina Herslinger and William Krasker.[29] These authors analyzed the performance of fourteen major hospital chains — six for-profit and eight nonprofit — in 1977 and 1981. Their sample consisted of 725 hospitals representing 90 percent of the hospital beds in the for-profit sector and 68 percent of the beds in the nonprofit sector in the U.S. After controlling for such factors as location, scope of services, the presence of teaching and research activities, care to indigent patients, quality of care, size, and price charged for services, they reported the following findings:

1. Although nonprofit hospitals receive more social subsidies than for-profits, they do not achieve better social results. They are not more accessible to the uninsured and medically indigent, nor do they price less aggressively. They are also more oriented toward short-term results than the for-profit hospitals are, replacing their plant and equipment much more slowly.
2. Nonprofits do, however, tend to maximize the welfare of the affiliated physicians, who are their main customers.

3. For-profit hospitals are more efficient than nonprofits, reinvest their earnings in new plant and equipment, and offer just as broad a range of services to a larger number of patients, including the indigent.
4. Nonprofit hospitals do not inevitably improve social welfare in their communities. The hospitals' professional staff capture many of the benefits
   inherent in the nonprofit form. This behavior is much less likely to occur
   in a for-profit organization subject to stock market discipline.

Health care may be different from ordinary commodities purchased
in the marketplace, but that does not mean that incentives do not matter
in health care markets or that the laws of supply and demand do not
apply there. Competitive markets provide powerful incentives to improve product or service quality constantly and to cut costs and hold
down prices, whereas nonprofit organizations — either private or governmental — are largely isolated from such competitive pressures. It is
not surprising, therefore, that for-profit hospitals are more efficient than
nonprofit ones. The health care sector could use more private enterprise, competition, and consumer choice, but the "new" public health
establishment adamantly opposes such proposals (as discussed further
in later chapters).

# 4

# The Radicalization of Public Health

*"The current government of Nicaragua has*
*given great priority to health services."*
*—American Public Health Association, 1983*

It was apparent by the mid-1970s that the American Public Health Association was being directed not by mainstream liberals, but by radicals who placed much greater reliance on political activism in the name of public health than had their predecessors. They routinely issued declarations of "solidarity" with communist tyrants around the world, notably in Cuba and Nicaragua. Essentially, as discussed in detail below, the APHA had evolved into an arm of the far left in American politics, using "public health" as a vehicle to promote socialism.

## Foreign Policy and Public Health

Consider: In the name of improving *American* public health, the APHA in the early 1980s strongly supported the communist Sandinista regime that had taken over the Nicaraguan government. The Nicaraguan communists were, after all, determined to impose socialism on the Nicaraguan economy, including the health care sector.

During the Cold War, both sides propagandized. One could never accept as truth anything that a communist government said without verification. But the APHA accepted the pronouncements of the Nicaraguan communists — especially the fact that they claimed to have improved health care. Of course, communist governments throughout the twentieth century claimed to have significantly increased resources for health care. Such is standard communist propaganda.

"The current government of Nicaragua has given great priority to health services," a 1983 APHA policy statement announced.[1] The communist government had claimed to have quadrupled health care expenditures and tripled health care personnel in just three years, and the APHA was impressed. It accordingly went on record as opposing the Reagan administration's effort to undermine the communist dictatorship by declaring it "feared" that "the Reagan Administration's newly stated policy ... to replace the current Nicaraguan government would reverse all these advances in health care."[2] The association then issued a resolution that "commends the efforts of the Nicaraguan government to improve the health status of the people" and formally condemned the Reagan administration's policy, urging it to "promote a policy of peace and harmony among all nations of Central America."[3] In 1984 the association again viewed "with alarm" the Reagan administration's "efforts at destabilization [sic] of the Nicaraguan Government," and condemned U.S. policy as "a threat to peace in Central America and the world."[4]

Peace and harmony were not things that the Nicaraguan communist government was promoting, as students of Central America at the time knew. And it was not a democratic government, as the APHA leadership must have known. After the Sandinistas took over the government by force of arms, they consolidated power and then immediately purged democratic sympathizers from the regime, announced that the government was communist, and began making frequent advisory trips to Cuba. Such actions belie the APHA's 1983 resolution in support of the Sandinistas, in which it declared belief "in the principle that the people of a nation should be allowed to determine their own form of government."[5]

The situation in Nicaragua was recently described by David Horowitz, formerly a celebrated intellectual leader of the Marxist left in America who in 1984 recanted his Marxist views in light of atrocities committed by his fellow Marxists around the globe. When Horowitz checked with his old comrades in the "New Left" political movement to find out who the Nicaraguan Sandinistas were, he "discovered them to be Marxist protégés of Castro who had announced their intention to turn Nicaragua into another Cuba," even though "In the twenty years of Castro's rule, Cuba had been transformed into a totalitarian state, its economy ruined by socialist plans, its jails filled with political dissenters."[6]

"Like Castro twenty years earlier," Horowitz writes, "the Sandinistas were able to seize power by concealing their Marxist agenda and leading a coalition of democrats against the Somoza regime.... But, once in power, the Sandinistas expelled the democrats from the ruling group and began implementing their Marxist design."[7]

When the Sandinistas were forced to hold elections, they were re-soundingly defeated, after destroying much of the Nicaraguan economy. "Every socialist state created by Marxists had been transformed into an economic sinkhole and a national prison. There were no exceptions," Horowitz reminds us.[8]

Such economic destruction reveals the lie in the propaganda that they were able to triple or quadruple the economic resources devoted to health care. The Nicaraguan people knew it was a lie, but the leadership of the APHA apparently did not discern this truth.

During the waning days of the Cold War the APHA often opposed U.S. foreign policy, which is not necessarily objectionable. It annually condemned the U.S. military establishment for challenging communism, was a participant in the "Nuclear Freeze Movement," which we now know was instigated and financed by the KGB, and condemned human rights abuses in various noncommunist countries, but said nothing about the human rights abuses in such places as Russia, Cuba, Romania, China, and other socialist countries. The APHA certainly was not wrong in condemning human rights abuses in noncommunist countries, but its bias in favor of communism raises serious questions about the APHA's sincerity.

The APHA leadership apparently viewed Cuba as a political and economic role model for the United States, especially with regard to health care. In 1977 it first issued a resolution opposing the U.S. embargo on trade with Cuba. The resolution was issued not because the APHA supports free trade — it does not, as discussed below. Rather, it was issued because the embargo "limits the access of the United States public to information about Cuba, including information on Cuba's accomplishments in public health."[9] If only Americans could learn of how wonderful life in Cuba was, the APHA evidently believed, they would be more likely to embrace socialism.

## Socialized Health Care: Improving Public Health?

The public health establishment did not restrict its agenda to foreign policy. Through the APHA, it has long endorsed central planning of the entire U.S. health care sector, including the total abolition of the private practice of medicine as we have known it. Each year for the past several decades the association has issued a resolution calling for the nationalization of health care in America. Typical of these resolutions is the one issued in 1976 calling for "comprehensive health care" provided "within a progressively financed, democratically controlled health system."[10] There would be no role for private health care providers or fee-for-service health care. Everything would be "democratically controlled," that is, controlled by government bureaucrats. Nationalized health care would supposedly "eliminate the unnecessary inflation of cost and utilization resulting from the current fee-for-service system."[11] It would also cover virtually anyone *in the world* who could make it to the United States, because it would cover residents of the U.S., Puerto Rico, the Northern Marianas, and U.S. Territories, *regardless of legal resident or immigration status*"[12] (emphasis added).

Privacy with regard to medical records would almost vanish under such a system, since the central planners would need this information for planning. Thus, the APHA "urges the President and the Congress to begin planning now for the development of an information system which will be required for a national health program."[13]

There should also be nationalized health insurance that would also require the complete abolition of the private health insurance industry. Furthermore, the association advocates the elimination of means testing — even millionaires would be covered by taxpayer-financed "insurance."

In case it is not possible to totally eliminate the private health care sector, "whatever private health care sector remains after the full implementation of a national health service must not be relieved of financially contributing to the latter."[14] Penalties and fines would be necessary to assure that everyone paid for nationalized health care, even if they didn't use it. Moreover, no part of private sector health care should be tax deductible, for that would undermine the goal of complete nationalization: "There should be no direct or indirect public subsidy to private purchase of health care under a national health service program."[15]

During the debate over the failed Clinton administration plan for nationalized medicine in the early 1990s Senator Phil Gramm (R-Tex.) frequently stated that "there's not enough money in the world to pay for the Clinton health plan." The senator holds a Ph.D. in economics and is a former Texas A&M economics professor. He understands the law of demand with respect to medical care, which says that if the explicit price of health care is set at zero, as it is with government-provided health care, then demand will be virtually unlimited. Everyone — rich and poor — will want more at a zero price. This explosion of demand will cause the total cost of health care to skyrocket to unprecedented levels, but such costs will be hidden in general tax revenues, at least for a while. It would likely require a doubling or tripling of the federal budget to pay for such a scheme. And, as is true of all government programs, it would be bound to become even *more* costly in the future than anyone today would anticipate. The APHA seems unconcerned with these economic facts and calls for "increasingly progressive taxation" to pay for it.[16]

Increasingly progressive taxation to finance such a scheme would be economically pernicious. "Progressive" taxation is designed specifically to punish disproportionately those who achieve the most economic success. In the United States the real engine of job creation is small business. While many of the largest corporations have been "downsizing," most of the millions of new jobs created annually are in relatively small businesses (who sometimes become very large themselves, as is the case of such companies as Apple Computer or Microsoft). Because most small business owners pay personal, not corporate income taxes, they are always punished severely by increasingly progressive taxation. Thus, progressive taxation will deter job creation and economic growth, diminishing our ability to pay for health care.

Every country with government-controlled health care has experienced an explosion of costs, which it then attempts to hold down with price controls, which are euphemistically referred to as "cost containment measures" by the APHA. As every economics student knows, price controls inevitably cause shortages, the deterioration of product or service quality, and the allocation of the short supply of goods or services by political rather than by economic criteria. Thus, in countries where there is nationalized medical care, such as Canada and Great Britain, there are serious problems with shortages and long waiting lists for various forms of health care, including surgery. Health care rationing is inevitable. Some people simply must be refused needed care, even if it shortens their lives.

In Canada, for example, the government has rationed health care resources by severely limiting access to medical technology. On a per capita basis, the United States has eight times more magnetic resonance imaging (MRI) units, seven times more radiation therapy units (for cancer treatment), six times more lithotripsy units (to destroy kidney stones and gallstones), and three times more open-heart surgery and cardiac catheterization units.[17] Physicians in British Columbia have taken out full-page newspaper ads warning that their patients' lives are in danger because the government has refused to purchase lifesaving medical technology.[18]

There are similar shortages of medical technology in Great Britain, another "role model" of nationalized medicine championed by the American public health establishment. A study by the Brookings Institution revealed that each year about 9,000 British kidney patients fail to receive renal dialysis or a kidney transplant and die as a result. About 15,000 cancer patients and 17,000 heart patients in Britain fail to receive the treatment that modern medicine can offer them, and about 7,000 elderly patients living in pain are denied hip replacements by the government health care bureaucracy.[19]

The denial of needed health care in these nationalized health care systems makes a mockery of the claim by its proponents that in such systems patients are granted "rights" to health care. In fact, thousands of citizens are routinely denied health care in those countries — health care that they would receive in the United States.

Another manifestation of the shortages caused by price controls in nationalized health care systems are the often long waiting lists for those in need of care. In Canada, patients must wait an average of 5.5 months for heart bypass surgery, 4.9 months for other open heart surgery, 5.7 months for hernia repair, and 3.7 months for a hysterectomy. In Ontario, patients wait up to six months for a CAT scan, up to a year for eye and orthopedic surgery, and up to two years for lithotripsy treatment, according to a survey by the U.S. General Accounting Office.[20]

Government bureaucracies are *inherently* inefficient — sometimes very much so — because of the absence of the competitive pressures that provide incentives for efficiency on the part of private, competitive firms. Because there is no bottom line, in an accounting sense, there really is no way to measure how "efficient" any government bureaucracy is at utilizing resources. But we do know that bureaucratic incentives tend to be rather perverse with regard to efficiency. Because government bureaucrats cannot be directly rewarded for cutting costs and saving taxpayers money, or by improving the quality of service, they are less inclined than for-profit businesses to strive to do so. Instead, they tend to advance personally by building a bigger empire and acquiring a larger budget. Even if a government bureaucrat's motives are pure—he or she truly only wants to serve the public interest—more resources must be acquired to achieve that objective.

Thus, there is constant pressure to acquire bigger and bigger budgets, which results in some rather bizarre behavior. For example, at the end of every budget year there is a spending binge, whether the agency needs to be spending the money or not. The reason is that if an agency budget is not depleted this year, it will be more difficult to acquire the same or a larger budget next year.

There is also an incentive to become excessively labor intensive since the road to promotion is more successfully traveled if one can demonstrate the ability to "manage" a larger staff. Moreover, it is very difficult to fire incompetent government employees because of civil service rules. Consequently, the way in which a government manager gets rid of incompetent or embarrassing employees is frequently to promote them to move them elsewhere in the system.

All these incentives lead to what Dr. Max Gammon, a British physician who observed nationalized health care in England for several decades, has labeled "Gammon's law" of bureaucracy. In a bureaucratic system, says Dr. Gammon, increases in expenditures will be matched by *reductions* in output. Such systems will act rather like "black holes" in the economic universe, simultaneously sucking in resources, and shrinking in terms of production.[21]

Gammon's research has shown how his "law" is in full force in England's nationalized health care sector. Nobel laureate economist Milton Friedman has inquired whether it might not apply to the United States as well. There is not full-blown health care socialism in the U.S., but there has been progressively more and more government control of the health care sector in the past fifty years, especially since the advent of Medicare and Medicaid in the 1960s.

Friedman examined "inputs and outputs" in the U.S. health care sector from 1929 — when hospitals were primarily private — until 1989 when, because of massive government subsidies to government and private "nonprofit" hospitals, the proprietary hospital sector had shrunk to about 15 percent of the total industry capacity. Because of this massive government takeover of the hospital industry, argues Friedman, we see "Gammon's law in full operation since the end of World War II."[22]

Before 1940, when the hospital sector was still mostly proprietary and driven by the profit motive, instead of bureaucratic incentives, additional expenditures on hospitals tended to result in more "output." The cost of hospital care per patient, adjusted for inflation, rose at about 5 percent per year from 1929 to 1940, whereas the number of occupied beds rose by 2.4 percent. Thus, costs rose only modestly and greater availability of hospital services was achieved.

The postwar situation was dramatically different, as the 1946

Hill-Burton Act authorized the expenditure of billions of dollars to construct government and nonprofit hospitals, leading to the decline of proprietary hospitals in the United States. With government dominating the hospital market in the postwar years, the number of hospital beds per one thousand population *fell* by more than one half and the occupancy rate dropped by an eighth. Costs, on the other hand, skyrocketed, as hospital personnel multiplied sevenfold and cost per patient-day, adjusted for inflation, rose twenty-six fold, from $21 in 1946 to $545 in 1989 (in constant 1989 dollars).

Part of this decline in hospital capacity can be explained by a healthier population, says Friedman, but improved health cannot fully explain the meteoric rise in hospital costs. Gammon's law was apparently at work as government-run hospitals became heavily bureaucratized. "Personnel per occupied bed, which had already doubled from 1946 to 1965, more than tripled from that level after 1965," while "cost per patient day, which had already more than tripled from 1946 to 1965, multiplied a further eightfold after 1965."[23] Because medicine has already "become in large part a socialist enterprise," concludes Friedman, "medicine in all its aspects has become subject to an ever more complex bureaucratic structure."[24]

By providing zero-price medical care to subsets of the U.S. population — the poor and the elderly — Medicare and Medicaid have caused an enormous rise in health care costs and have contributed greatly to the bureaucratization of health care. Yet the APHA's health care agenda would compel the *entire* population of the country, not just these two subsets, to participate in a zero-(explicit)-price health care system with no means testing. Such a program would create a huge bureaucracy. But, since public health bureaucrats would be running the system, *they* would benefit from it financially and in terms of political power, even if the American public did not.

## Bureaucratic Bungling Abroad

Despite the praise given nationalized health care by the public health establishment, the truth is that it is no more efficient than government-run programs in general. Government-run health care, like government-run post offices, schools, and most everything else, is inefficient and excessively costly. The notion that employing large numbers of *additional* federal government bureaucrats to run the health care industry *monopoly* would improve effi-

ciency is absurd. Yet, that is the argument of those advocating nationalized health care.

But as the economists John Goodman and Gerald Musgrave observed after surveying nationalized health care worldwide,
"[G]overnment-run hospitals in other countries are disastrously inefficient. It is not unusual to find a modern laboratory and an anti-
quated radiology department in the same hospital. Nor is it unusual
to find one hospital with a nursing shortage near another with a nursing surplus.... Moreover, even when specific inefficiencies are
acknowledged, it is often impossible to eliminate them because of
political pressures."[25] Even the best British hospitals do not keep com-
puterized records, so that it is impossible to gain accurate information on just how costly they are. And in terms of organizational skills
and managerial efficiency, the government-run hospitals of other countries "cannot begin to match hospitals run by Hospital Corporation of
America, Humana, or American Medical International."[26]

The inefficiencies in all government-run health care industries are
not just quirks that can be fixed by "experts" with advanced degrees in
public health. They are *inherent* because of the laws of politics. The
incentives in politics guarantee that nationalized health care is no more
efficient than government-run schooling or postal delivery. It would
mean receiving care from a government agency with all the efficiency
of the U.S. Postal Service and all the compassion of the IRS.

The proponents of nationalized health care always argue that it
would be more "equitable" than in a system driven by market incentives. But Goodman convincingly explained why the gross inefficiencies of the British National Health Service are inherent in a comprehensive study of that system published in 1980.[27] In England and in
all other countries where health care is almost 100 percent nationalized, the decision to spend on health services — and where to spend
it — is inevitably political. Consequently, per-capita spending on
health care varies significantly across Great Britain for political reasons. It tends to be allocated more to those regions where there are
more votes and campaign contributions, regardless of health care needs
of the population. One study found that people in Great Britain's highest social class (and also its most effective political "class") received
40 percent more medical care (in relation to their need for it) than
people in the lowest social class.[28] In general, according to Goodman
and Musgrave, when health care is rationed by government, "the poor
are pushed to the rear of the waiting line."[29]

One marked difference between the British and American health care systems is the British emphasis on "caring" versus curing, according to Goodman. One reason for this difference, notes economist Mary-Ann Rozbicki, is that "caring" wins more votes than curing does: "In weighing the choice between a more comfortable life for the millions of aged or early detection and treatment of the far fewer victims of dread diseases, [British National Health Service bureaucrats] have favored the former.... The sheer numbers involved on each side of the equation would tend to dictate these choices by government officials in a democratic society."[30]

Moreover, British citizens may not seem to care about this allocation of health care resources because they are what public choice economists call "rationally ignorant" about health care services. People have fewer incentives to inquire about alternative services when they are served by a government-run monopoly. Indeed, what would be the point of inquiring at all about alternatives if such alternatives are illegal or nonexistent? Thus, because they are ignorant of the benefits of alternative patterns of health care benefits, they acquiesce in the current system.

Another feature of nationalized health care — and of all government-run activities — is an inherent shortsightedness with regard to capital expenditure. All politicians are primarily motivated to please a majority of voters *just prior to the next election*, which is never more than a few years off. A successful politician will strive to dispense government-financed benefits on his or her constituents now, while disguising or deferring the costs to the future, perhaps even decades later if the current spending is financed by long-term debt.

As a consequence of this political preference for short-term over long-term spending, the British National Health Service suffers from a debilitating reduction of its capital stock. As of 1980 over 50 percent of the hospital beds in Britain were in buildings built in the nineteenth century and there were fewer hospital beds in the country than there were in 1945.[31]

By contrast, in competitive private markets, those who make successful long-term decisions will be rewarded with higher profits. Shortsightedness in investment planning is penalized in private competitive markets, but it is "rewarded" in politics. As British economists John and Sylvia Jewkes noted about the British health care system: "Governments followed the line of least resistance. They laid emphasis on those medical items which constituted pressing day-to-day demand, yielded their results quickly and with some certainty, made something of a public splash and conformed with the doctrine of equality. Conversely, they tended to neglect those items where spending would bring only slowly maturing results, where economy would not be quickly noticed and therefore would be less likely to arouse public opposition."[32]

Another inherent feature of politicized health care is that it tends to benefit special interest groups first and foremost. Thus, a common criticism of the British system is that the industry "exists for its own sake, in the interest of the producer groups that make it up. The welfare of patients is a random by-product, depending on how conflicts between the groups and between them and government happen to shake down at any particular time."[33]

In light of the earlier discussion, it is interesting to note what a Nicaraguan physician, Dr. Roberto Calderon, has said of Nicaragua's nationalized health care system under the Sandinista regime. During a decade of practicing medicine while the Sandinistas were in power Dr. Calderon came to the following conclusions about nationalized health care:

- The patient can never choose his or her doctor; the bureaucratic process makes all the important decisions. There's little room for free choice — for switching from one doctor to another, for instance — because everyone has to go by the bureaucrats' rules. Too much freedom for the patients makes life more difficult for the bureaucrats, so that freedom is all but absent.
- The doctor cannot choose the patient, either, because assignments are determined by rigid bureaucratic rules. Referring a patient to another (better qualified or more highly specialized) doctor is considered to be an "unnecessary complication" that imposes further paperwork on the bureaucrats.
- The doctor gets paid a fixed amount at the end of each month regardless of his or her performance, a prescription for high cost and poor performance.
- Doctors are given no incentives to develop a good bedside manner because they are under such great pressure to treat large numbers of patients.
- The system simply does not work. Patients don't get well because of the previous four points.
- There were massive shortages of just about everything, from physicians and nurses to equipment and medicines. Many people were put on long waiting lists for emergency surgery and died before being treated.[34]

What Dr. Calderon observed are, of course, features of nationalized health care everywhere.

## Statistical Murder

Professor John Graham of Harvard University's School of Public Health is one of the nation's top experts in risk analysis — the science of evaluating the health risks involved in various kinds of behaviors, from smoking to driving without seatbelts, to living in poverty. There are many public health professionals like Professor Graham who believe that public health dollars ought to be spent efficiently — that is, the most money ought to be spent in areas where it will save or prolong the most lives. An expenditure of say, $1 billion to save a single life would be "inefficient" if that same sum could be spent elsewhere to save 100 or 1,000 lives.

This is the essence of benefit/cost analysis as it is applied to risky behavior and its effects on health. The idea is *not* for scientific "experts" to pass judgment on whether or not someone's life is worth saving. Risk or benefit/cost analysis is employed to assist policymakers in answering the question: If X dollars are to be spent to improve public health, how can they be most efficiently allocated in a way that is most beneficial to public health? It recognizes that because all resources — including public health resources — are scarce, *tradeoffs are pervasive*. Spending a public health dollar for one purpose means that dollar is not spent somewhere else. The objective of benefit/cost analysis is to assist in maximizing the public health benefits of government's public health programs.

When interviewed by ABC News television reporter John Stossel, Professor Graham said that if a certain amount of money was spent to save one life when it could have instead been spent to save 100 lives, then that's a case of "statistical murder." It is statistical because you cannot pinpoint a single life lost. There was no malign motive, just inept or *inefficient* decision making.

There are numerous examples of public health dollars being wasted, with little or no public health benefits. It is this kind of spending that economists and public health professionals like Graham refer to when they criticize misguided government health regulation. They are not opposed to government expenditures or regulations to improve public health. They *are* opposed to *wasteful* public health spending — spending that could have produced more public health benefits than it did. Thus, they are critical of such government policies as the mandate to remove asbestos from public school buildings in America, a $5 billion per year industry, despite the fact that scientists now know that the kind of asbestos used in insulation in public buildings is harmless if left alone. Surely, that $5 billion annually could produce more health benefits if spent elsewhere.

They are critical of many of the scientifically phony health scares, typified by the claim several years ago that the chemical Alar, a growth regulator sprayed on apples, could cause cancer. The apple industry reportedly lost $250 million and apple processors lost another $125 million. The scare turned out to be phony, however, as the "research" that led to it was discredited. The "researchers" apparently fed mice the equivalent of 19,000 quarts of apple juice every day for a lifetime to make them become ill.[35]

In late 1996 the U.S. Environmental Protection Agency proposed new clean air standards limiting ground-level ozone that its own science advisers said would not be significantly more protective of public health despite imposing billions of dollars of costs annually on consumers and business owners. The agency estimated the costs to be as much as $6.3 billion annually. It said the new rules could help reverse the rising incidence of asthma — especially in children — even though the incidence of asthma has risen while air quality has been steadily *improving*.[36] Thus, any health benefits to children would be small, at best, although the costs would likely exceed the total amount that the federal government spends on child health through the National Heart, Lung and Blood Institute, the National Institute of Child Health and Human Development, and the National Institute of Environmental Health Science.

These funds would obviously improve public health more significantly if spent in other ways. Furthermore, the costs of the regulations themselves reduce public health, for "the rule would make goods and services more expensive, causing disposable family income to decline. It is widely recognized that health improves as family incomes rise."[37]

The U.S. Office of Management and Budget recently found that every $9 million to $12 million decline in aggregate personal income is associated with one "statistical death." Using these figures, combined with the EPA's own estimates of the costs of its proposal, it has been estimated that the "clean air" proposal will result in as many as 700 deaths each year. Economists Wendy Gramm and Susan Dudley believe that the EPA has understated the cost estimates. Their higher estimate of costs leads to the conclusion that the EPA proposal could result in as many as 7,000 additional deaths — cases of "statistical murder"— each year.[38]

Not all public health professionals believe, as does Graham, that public health dollars should be allocated in a way that saves the most lives. Some EPA employees obviously do not, nor do the most extreme segments of the Washington, D.C.-based environmentalist movement, which seem more determined to punish "capitalists" than to improve public health. And the American Public Health Association has also officially stated its opposition to the use of benefit/cost analysis in regulatory decision making, recommending that its members develop testimony on federal, state, and local legislation, send letters to legislators, and organize "grass-roots letter-writing campaigns" to "prohibit requirements that regulation must always demonstrate a positive benefit-cost ratio and forbid decision-making on health-related regulation solely on the basis of cost-benefit analysis."[39]

Essentially, the public health establishment denies that resources are scarce and that trade-offs are inevitable. It endorses the view that consumers' pockets are bottomless when it comes to government-imposed costs. It also apparently denies what every economist knows: By reducing the rate of economic growth, government regulation can be harmful to public health. In doing so it makes it all the more likely that government's regulatory policy will commit statistical murder.

## (Mis)Pronouncements on Economic Policy

The APHA makes numerous statements regarding the relationship between economic conditions and public health. It notes correctly that higher unemployment rates are usually accompanied by more severe public health problems, even including a higher incidence of suicide. But the policies it recommends tend only to make these problems worse.

For example, in 1995 the association issued a formal policy statement on "Full Employment and Public Health" noting the negative health effects of unemployment.[40] So far, so good. But then it based its policy recommendations on a number of demonstrably false assumptions, such as the assertion that the Federal Reserve "has not been effective in dealing with the threat of inflation."[41] As of 1995 — when this statement was written — inflation was all but nonexistent and the unemployment rate was about 5 percent, most of which was voluntary unemployment, that is, people not working because they are in the process of changing jobs.

In keeping with its fundamental belief that there is an economic free lunch, the APHA recommended that the federal government implement a policy "ensuring employment guaranteed at a living wage to every adult man or woman who is unable to find adequately remunerative work in the normal labor market."[42] Such government employment should include health insurance benefits equivalent to the generous package given to federal bureaucrats, "safe and healthy working conditions," and even "quality childcare services." And unemployment insurance benefits should be increased as well.

Such a policy pronouncement reveals a complete lack of rudimentary economic understanding. As mentioned in chapter 3, it is impossible for government spending programs to "create jobs." Government spending programs can only *reallocate* the kind of jobs that exist — more government jobs, fewer private-sector jobs. The money that must go to pay for the jobs must be extracted from the private sector one way or another, thereby depressing economic conditions there and thus actually increasing unemployment. The best government can do to encourage job creation, as discussed in chapter 3, is to create an environment that protects private property rights and enforces contracts while minimizing the tax and regulatory burden on the populace, permitting free trade, and eliminating regulatory barriers to employment, such as occupational licensing laws that often are designed as barriers to entry in employment.

Because many democratic governments have failed to control their spending and routinely run huge budget deficits, they are inclined to resort to mandating employment "benefits" provided by employers. One such mandate is what the APHA calls a "living wage." In some cities, such as Baltimore, Maryland, governments have mandated that employers doing business with them must pay unskilled workers at least a "living wage" of about $10 per hour. The problem, however, is that some unskilled, inexperienced workers are not yet capable of producing $10 an hour worth of goods or services for a business. Consequently, the mandated "living wage" prices them out of employment. An employer might be willing to hire them at say, $8 an hour, but not $10.

The APHA's recommendation of a "full employment policy" that includes child care, generous insurance benefits, and other perks would also cause significantly higher unemployment. It simply would drive up the cost of hiring labor; at a higher (government-mandated) price employers will hire fewer people. If the policy were to be implemented through a government spending program, it is obvious that fewer jobs could be handed out by government (which does, after all, have a fixed budget each year) than the private sector would create if each job is more expensive. The more money that is spent on government jobs, the more that is extracted from the private sector through taxation, causing higher unemployment there. By fueling big government the public health establishment shrinks the private sector, the sole source of genuine job creation. Such policies would, in other words, cause higher unemployment and the higher incidence of public health problems that accompany it.

On the important issue of international trade, the APHA also advocates policies that will destroy jobs and make the country poorer. It essentially embraces the political agendas of the AFL-CIO and the extreme environmentalists with regard to trade. In 1994 it issued resolutions supporting these two interest groups' positions on international trade agreements that: (1) Every country that is a partner to a free-trade agreement must agree to an "upward" harmonization of labor market regulation so that all countries have the level of regulation that the most heavily regulated country has; and (2) a similar "upward harmonization" should occur with regard to environmental regulation.[43]

As discussed in chapter 3, excessive regulation reduces economic prosperity. What the APHA endorses is the "upward harmonization" of economic problems caused by regulation. Labor unions realize that many of the regulations they favor render American businesses less competitive in international markets, so they advocate burdening less developed trading partners, such as Mexico, with the same economically burdensome regulations to reduce international competition. Such "harmonization," then, is specifically aimed at reducing the economic growth and opportunities in foreign countries, all in the name of improving "public health" internationally!

The APHA recommendation urges that all trade agreements also be influenced by a coalition of special interest groups, such as the International Labor Organization, to "assure" upward harmonization of government regulation, and also supports numerous "studies" of the possible ill-health effects of international trade.

The public health establishment's position on international trade, therefore, is to support a form of veiled protectionism. As such, it will make Americans poorer and create higher unemployment. Freedom of commerce always enhances the wealth of nations and provides additional economic opportunities. Protectionism benefits relatively small special interest groups — at least temporarily — usually at much greater expense to the rest of the nation in terms of lost economic opportunities.

On most economic issues, the public health establishment urges more taxes, more regulation, and more government control of private-sector businesses and consumers. It rarely, if ever, advocates economic freedom.

The APHA is so paternalistic that it even urges the federal government to ban the manufacture of toy guns and supports government-funded "efforts directed at parents on the risks of confusion between toy and real guns."[45] It also wants the government to censure any television programs that the APHA and its political allies believe might have negative health consequences, particularly on "children and young people." Such policies implicitly assume that parents and adults have little or no responsibility for their children and that the federal government must play a much larger role in raising them.

## Public Health's Animus Towards Business

Perhaps the best example of the American public health establishment's anti-business perspective is the APHA's 1981 policy statement that "endorses a boycott of all products and services of the Nestlé Corporation."[46] In the late 1970s Nestlé, the world's largest producer of baby formula, was accused of being responsible for the deaths of Third World babies where mothers had mixed the company's infant formula with contaminated water. The APHA joined the Infant Formula Action Coalition (INFACT), which included about 100 organizations.

The Nestlé boycott and the propaganda campaign surrounding it was characterized by harsh, anti-corporate rhetoric and Marxist slogans. One INFACT activist, Mark Ritchie, explained that the main purpose of the boycott was not to improve infant health in Third World countries, but "to link the capitalist system — and the way it organizes our lives — to people's very personal experiences."[47]

The organizers of the boycott announced to the media that ten million Third World babies were starving because of "the heartless, money-hungry activities of powerful multinational companies."[48] But Derrick B. Aellife, the chief organizer of the boycott, admitted to *Newsweek* that the figure of 10 million was only "symbolic" and not based on fact.[49] James Grant, the executive director of UNICEF, later offered a much lower figure — one million — but also admitted that this was only a guess.

The main claims made by the INFACT coalition were that corporate advertising contributed greatly to a mother's decision to bottle feed; there had been a dramatic decline in breast feeding in developing countries; bottle-fed babies come largely from the poorest families; and bottle-fed babies have higher disease rates than those who are breast fed. But when asked about these propositions at a Congressional hearing, INFACT witnesses simply didn't know anything about breast-feeding habits in third world countries.[50] It was also revealed at the hearing that the few studies that existed showed that poor women tend to rely *more* on breast feeding than more affluent mothers, contrary to INFACT's assertions. Investigative journalist Carol Adelman surveyed what evidence existed at the time and concluded:

> Of the four studies most frequently cited to support the key assumption ... two had nothing to do with the assumption. Of the remaining two studies, one did not scientifically examine the question and demonstrated results that conflicted with the author's opinions. The other did show an increase in breast feeding but did not prove that formula advertising was the single or even major cause."[51]

It was eventually revealed that what INFACT wanted was not an end to the use of infant formula, but an end to the selling of the formula by private enterprises — what it called "de-marketing." At a 1979 Congressional hearing, Edward Baer, an INFACT board member, cited as a role model of infant formula supply communist Algeria, where the importation and sale of infant formula was in the hands of a government-run monopoly. When it was pointed out that the importation of infant formula into Algeria had risen from 2.5 million cans in 1976 to 12 million in 1979 — the kind of thing INFACT had condemned when Nestlé was selling the formula — Baer replied that it didn't bother him at all because it was taking place under governmental control.[52] Capitalist infant formula was dangerous, according to Mr. Baer, but infant formula when sold by government was safe.

The U.S. government did not sign onto the United Nations code that would limit the marketing of infant formula by private enterprises in developing countries, ceding much of the business to governmental monopolies there. But the American public health establishment supported the boycott and the code. It simply does not want the private sector to play any role whatsoever in the delivery of health care services, and it takes any chance it gets to limit the domain of voluntarism and free choice in health care while expanding the reach of government.

# 5

# Is the Second Amendment Hazardous to Public Health?

*"Guns are a virus that must be eradicated.... Get rid of the guns, get rid of the bullets, and you get rid of deaths."*
*—Dr. Katherine Christoffel,*
*National Center for Injury Prevention and Control*

The modus operandi of the "new public health" was clearly defined in an article published in the August 1996 issue of *Health Education Quarterly*, which was widely distributed by the Office of Communications at the Centers for Disease Control and Prevention (CDC), as an example of what CDC employees ought to be doing with their careers.[1] The article explains how "media advocacy" is fundamentally different from the traditional use of the media to provide health information to the public. The traditional approach is based on the idea that public health professionals should, among other things, disseminate information that the public can then use to improve their health, for example, refrain from smoking, eat right, exercise regularly, drink moderately, and so on. Individuals are free to use the information or not; many of them will use the advice and will benefit from it.

According to this traditional view, health is defined primarily as the absence of disease, and disease is associated with known risk factors, which can be controlled to an extent by individual behavior. Thus, the key to controlling these risk factors is the provision of knowledge and skills to the individual. Freely choosing individuals who benefit from health care information can make for a healthier society.

In sharp contrast, the "new public health" is premised on the notion that improved health does *not* come from individual choices regarding lifestyle, medication, and so on, but from "participation in the public policy process."[2] Thus, "policy advocacy skills for creating social change must be provided to community groups *rather than, for example, pro-*

53

*viding individuals with skills so that they can make better personal choices* (emphasis added)."[3] For example, "rather than distributing nutrition pamphlets with low-fat recipes, political pressure is placed on [local government] planning commissions to approve fewer alcohol outlets and more produce stores."[4]

The objective of "media advocacy," as used in "the new public health" movement, is nothing less than "to rethink the foundation of basic values on which society is based" and to engage in the process of "redesigning society" through the use of political coercion.[5] The objective, in other words, is to *lobby* for government control and regulation of behavior leading to polices such as those described in the two previous chapters.

The hallmark of this new approach to "media advocacy" is intolerance of freedom of individual choice — even of the kind of choices that affect no one but the individual decision maker. For example, practitioners of the new public health are not content with educating Americans about the dangers of smoking; they must ban smoking, depriving adults of freedom of choice. These paternalistic professionals will try to get the government to *force* stubborn American smokers to live as the professionals think they should live. Sometimes "even education ... is not sufficient to create significant changes in important health behaviors over an extended period of time."[6]

If people continue to smoke, eat fast food, and exercise only irregularly, despite their full knowledge of the health risks involved in such behavior, then one can only assume that these individuals have assessed the *trade-offs* facing them and decided that they will gain more happiness by continuing to live as they have been. The new public health, however, seeks to direct the entire public health profession in the direction of using governmental coercion to prohibit individuals from making their own lifestyle choices. The new public health movement is all about coercing the public through governmental action, as the next several chapters will reveal.

## The Public Health Campaign for Gun Control

Based on often flimsy evidence, the new public health frequently takes the position that it has discovered THE TRUTH about various policy issues, that there can be no question about its interpretation of that "truth," and that only fools or those with hidden agendas would resist instituting that "truth" as the law of the land.

One example of this phenomenon is the movement's government-funded lobbying for gun control laws. There is anything but universal — or even majority — agreement over the desirability of such laws, but public health professionals are using tax dollars to try to impose such laws on the nation.

As a case in point, the CDC sponsors "violence prevention conferences" which focus not so much on health and medical issues, but on the development of lobbying techniques. One conference brochure, for example, highlights sessions on "media advocacy training," "media literacy," and other tools of the trade for lobbyists, not traditional public health professionals.[7] The CDC also finances the publication of an "Injury Prevention Network Newsletter" which addresses itself to "Advocates" (i.e., lobbyists).[8] The newsletter contains much useful information for women who are the victims of domestic violence, but it also argues that "we should start thinking about firearms as we do any other hazardous material — and that is by going to the sources, just as we go to smoke stacks as the source of pollution."[9]

The Spring 1995 newsletter reported on a government- sponsored symposium on "Articulating Guns and Violence as a Women's Issue" and advised "advocates" to "put gun control on the agenda of your civic or professional organization"; "oppose repeal of the [federal] assault weapons ban"; lobby for "restricting ammunition availability"; increase "restrictions on issuance of concealed weapons permits"; lobby to "allow cities and counties to regulate firearms"; organize "a picket at gun manufacturing sites"; and encourage local police to prohibit "officers from recommending that citizens buy guns for protection."[10]

Although these messages and the conference they were developed at were funded by the CDC's National Center for Injury Prevention and Control (NCIPC), ostensibly for "firearm injury research," there is no research here on firearm injuries, only tips on how to become more effective at lobbying. The presumption is that there is no need at all for any further research on the effects of gun availability — the only "problem" is how to get more laws passed banning gun ownership.

Congress recognized in 1996 that the CDC was illegally funding lobbying seminars for gun control advocates under the guise of "injury research," so it added the following rider to the CDC's appropriation bill: "None of the funds made available for injury prevention and control at the Centers for Disease Control and Prevention may be used to advocate or promote gun control."[11] But Congress has passed literally hundreds of such laws over the years. The laws are simply flouted by both government agencies and federally funded nonprofit organizations, as we showed in our 1985 book, *Destroying Democracy: How Government Funds Partisan Politics*, and again in 1998 in *CancerScam: Diversion of Federal Cancer Funds to Politics*.[12]

In response to Congress's attempt to enforce existing laws prohibiting tax-funded politics the *American Journal of Public Health* ran an editorial comment by noted gun control advocate Arthur Kellermann of Emory University. Kellermann decried Congress's action, declaring it to be "arguably the most egregious" example of special-interest influence in American history (presumably referring to the influence on Congress of the National Rifle Association).[13] Nevertheless, Kellermann forecast that the "public health community" would eventually demonize firearm manufacturers as successfully as it had demonized cigarette companies, paving the way for even more restrictions on firearm ownership. Interestingly, when Kellermann was once asked by a *San Francisco Examiner* reporter if he would want his own wife to have access to a firearm if she were attacked he answered: "If that were my wife [being attacked], would I want her to have a .38 Special in her hand? Yeah."[14]

The new public health movement essentially argues for eliminating guns by governmental fiat. As Dr. Katherine Christoffel of the HELP Network argued at a CDC-funded "strategy conference" for gun control advocates in 1995, "Guns are a virus that must be eradicated. We need to immunize ourselves against them.... Get rid of the cigarettes, get rid of the secondhand smoke, and you get rid of lung disease. It's the same with guns. Get rid of the guns, get rid of the bullets, and you get rid of deaths."[15] Presumably, according to Dr. Christoffel's logic, the same can be said of knives, rocks, automobiles, and all other inanimate objects that "cause" death.

The NCIPC's "research" is not without its critics in the medical profession. Dr. William C. Waters of Doctors for Integrity in Policy Research wrote a letter to U.S. Senator Arlen Specter (R-Pa.) complaining that

> We believe that the NCIPC fails to do its job because of unscientific bias.... First is the overt political activism of the NCIPC staff and their federally-funded researchers. Second ... is that there seems to be a tacit assumption — perhaps even a foundational concept — among many public health researchers that firearm prohibition/control provides a ready solution to many of society's ills. We believe that this view is expressed in the NCIPC's approach to the problem of violence in human societies ... and is often performed using abysmally poor methodology.... There seems to be a tendency on the part of those defending the NCIPC to simply reiterate figures depicting the problem of firearms violence/injury as justification for the agency's existence.[16]

## Paternalism, Elitism, and Intolerance

Gun control advocates in the public health community don't believe Americans can be trusted to purchase firearms for their own protection. They apparently think that it is all right for *them* to own firearms, but the rest of us should be prohibited by law from gun ownership. They are also intolerant of opposing opinions and frequently wage fierce political campaigns to keep others — especially other health professionals — from questioning their "evidence," which is frequently based on questionable science.

A case in point is the experience of Dr. Miguel Faria, a professor of neurosurgery at Mercer Medical School in Macon, Georgia. Dr. Faria was, until 1995, the editor of the *Journal of the Medical Association of Georgia*. A neurosurgeon who had spent incalculable hours treating victims of gunshot wounds, Dr. Faria "was researching the topic of violence" and "came to the inescapable conclusion and appalling reality that the medical literature on guns and self-protection had failed to objectively discuss both sides of the issue."[17] So Dr. Faria devoted part of an issue of his journal to a series of articles on firearms and gun violence by medical and nonmedical authors (i.e., legal and constitutional scholars) whom he expected to come down on both sides of the issue — exactly the kind of thing a scientific journal published at a medical school ought to do.

An article by Dr. Edgar Suter and thirty-seven co-authors, mostly physicians, raised serious questions about the work of Arthur Kellermann by showing that between twenty-five and seventy-five lives are *saved* by *defensive* uses of guns for every life that is lost because of a gun. After surveying the writings of the American founding fathers, legal scholar and nationally known gun expert David Kopel also stated in the journal that "the Second Amendment was plainly intended to guarantee the right of individuals to own guns."[18]

This was too much for the gun control advocates in the "new" public health movement to bear. As described in the *Augusta Chronicle*, "Almost immediately, vicious public attacks on Faria commenced — which caused [the Medical Association of Georgia's] executive committee to force the editor's resignation."[19] Dr. Faria was told that he made too many doctors "uncomfortable" by publishing articles on both sides of the gun control issue. The Georgia physicians were apparently intimidated by the editorial writers at the *Atlanta Journal and Consti-*

*tution*, who editorialized against Dr. Faria and mocked the idea that the Second Amendment to the U.S. Constitution defends gun ownership.

Even the *New England Journal of Medicine* weighed in on the issue with an ad hominem editorial by Dr. Jerome P. Kassirer, who has published several CDC-funded studies critical of gun ownership. Instead of discussing *any* of the substance of the articles published under Dr. Faria's editorship, Dr. Kassirer devoted his editorial to innuendo that asked if Dr. Faria might not be a secret plant of the National Rifle Association. He offered no evidence of any such connection, but the mere accusation, appearing in such a prestigious publication apparently sullied Dr. Faria's reputation and sent a strong message to any other physicians who might consider voicing less politically correct views of the gun control issue.

Anyone trained in the scientific method, as Dr. Kassirer obviously was, knows that personal attacks are irrelevant and inappropriate. It is the logic and evidence presented by researchers that is worthy of comment. The pro-gun control lobby in the medical profession is heavily funded by the CDC which, like every other government bureaucracy, is interested in expanding its budget and power. An honest, objective, scientific debate must be premised on the notion that the source of funding for pro-gun control research is irrelevant; it is the research itself that should be scrutinized.

Dr. Faria claims he sincerely believes that, based on existing evidence, gun control will end up costing more lives than it saves, and denies having any connection to the gun lobby. Nevertheless, his views are sure to be dismissed by practitioners of the new public health who view guns and bullets as "virulent pathogens" and who crusade for gun control laws.

## Is the Evidence on Gun Control Really That One-Sided?

Judging from the reaction of the public health profession to the mere mention, in a small medical journal published in Macon, Georgia, that there might possibly exist two sides to the gun control debate, one would get the impression that the research is overwhelmingly in favor of the notion that gun control laws work, that they save lives, and that they unequivocally improve public health. Certainly this is what one would expect in light of the fact that the U.S. Public Health Service has, since 1979, announced the goal of reducing the number of handguns in private ownership, starting with a 25 percent reduction by the year 2000.

In reality there is considerable evidence that gun control laws themselves are a source of violence, bloodshed, and death because they make it more difficult (in some cases impossible) for law-abiding citizens to acquire guns for purposes of self-defense.

San Francisco civil liberties attorney Don B. Kates, Atlanta physician William Waters, and Henry E. Schaffer, a professor of genetics and biomathematics at North Carolina State University, recently surveyed some of the most current and influential research by public health gun control advocates, such as Arthur Kellermann, and have found that much of the research has been thoroughly discredited, although that fact is rarely reported in the news media.[20]

Kates, Waters, and Schaffer found that "one hallmark of the public health literature on guns is a tendency to ignore contrary scholarship,"[21] and this literature often ignores scholarship in the fields of criminology and sociology if it does not support the public health movement's political agenda. Moreover, much of the research is published by people with no background in criminology or other relevant fields, but are individuals with degrees in public health.

Perhaps the most glaring omission in the public health literature is an almost complete absence of any mention of a book by Gary Kleck, a Florida State University criminologist, entitled *Point Blank: Guns and Violence in America* or of John Lott's book, *More Guns, Less Crime*. Kleck's encyclopedic work "assembles strong evidence against the notion that reducing gun ownership is a good way to reduce violence" and persuasively argues that "guns are used in self-defense up to three times as often as they are used to commit crimes."[22]

When CDC-funded public health gun control researchers do cite contrary evidence they frequently get it wrong, even stating conclusions that are the opposite of what the researchers they are citing actually concluded. For example, Arthur Kellermann frequently cites a book entitled *Under the Gun*, by sociologists James Wright and Peter Rossi, as supporting gun control. But what these authors actually say in their book is that "there is no persuasive evidence that supports this view [pro-gun control]."[23]

Kellermann is also fond of citing a 1992 *Journal of Psychiatry* article that allegedly says that limiting access to firearms would reduce the number of suicides, even though the article clearly concludes the opposite: People who don't have guns find other ways to kill themselves if they are so disposed.

Kellermann — and many other CDC-funded researchers — refuses to share his data with others, a breach of one of the most elementary canons of the scientific method. In economics, for example, it is routine for the authors of academic journal articles either to include their data as an appendix to the article or to put in writing that their data are available for the asking. Some economics journals even require one or the other as a condition of publication. So, when Kellermann asserted in a 1993 *New England Journal of Medicine* article that keeping a gun in the home "nearly triples" the likelihood that someone in the household will be killed with the gun, no one was able to scrutinize the claim, which received massive publicity in the media.

One of the biggest flaws in many of the CDC-funded gun control studies is that they confuse correlation with causation. For example, a Kellermann study purported to find that higher suicide rates are correlated with a greater predominance of gun ownership within a community. But as Kates, Schaffer, and Waters point out, merely finding a statistical correlation

> does not prove that having a gun in the house raises the risk of suicide.... Perhaps gun ownership in this sample was associated with personality traits that were, in turn, related to suicide or perhaps people who had contemplated suicide bought a gun for that reason. To put the association in perspective, it's worth noting that living alone and using illicit drugs were both better predictors of suicide than gun ownership was. That does not necessarily mean that living alone or using drugs leads to suicide.[24]

CDC-funded gun control research simply ignores a large body of data that contradict its pro-gun control position. For example, "in the 25 years from 1968 to 1992, American gun ownership increased almost 135 percent (from 97 million to 222 million), with handgun ownership rising more than 300 percent. These huge increases coincided with a two-thirds *decline* in accidental gun fatalities."[25]

The most likely reasons for the decline in accidental gun deaths are the pervasive gun safety programs of the National Rifle Association and other civic organizations, along with a substitution of handguns for shotguns for purposes of safety and self-defense. Meanwhile, the Centers for Disease Control ignores such facts because they contradict its preconceived ideas.

Another flaw in the CDC's gun control studies is that they all attempt to show statistical correlations with the mere number of guns, ignoring how the guns are distributed within the population — who has them, and for what purpose. Thus, gun control laws that limit overall gun availability without targeting the criminals who are the ones who use them illegitimately are bound to be ineffective and counterproductive.

This alleged correlation between the total number of guns owned by the populace and gun violence is the basis of what is called the "instrumentality theory" of guns and violence, which is the keystone of the CDC-funded gun control movement. The instrumentality theory at first seems commonsensical. It asserts that the availability of guns makes whatever crimes that are committed more deadly than they would otherwise be. Like so many other misguided and ill-informed theories of crime, this one was promoted by former U.S. Attorney General Ramsey Clark in his 1970 book, *Crime in America*.[26]

But as Northwestern University law professor Daniel D. Polsby has written, the instrumentality theory has "virtually collapsed" in light of voluminous contradicting evidence — evidence that is ignored by the CDC.[27] Among the "nagging anomalies" listed by Professor Polsby are the following:

- A 1979 study by University of Illinois sociologists David Bordua and Alan Lizotte showed that where guns were found in the greatest percentage of households, the rate of gun crimes was *lower*, and vice versa.
- The Chicago Metropolitan Crime Survey replicated Bordua and Lizotte's results as recently as 1996.
- Survey research shows conclusively that guns are used defensively and lawfully much more often than they are used in crimes. Almost 2.5 million crimes are thwarted each year in the U.S. by ordinary citizens brandishing firearms, according to a survey conducted by Florida State University criminologist Gary Kleck.[28]
- Contrary to popular belief guns are *less* available than they were thirty years ago, when handguns, shotguns, rifles, and ammunition could be bought over-the-counter at almost any hardware store. Guns could also be purchased by almost anyone, sight unseen, by mail order. Firearms have been *less* available since the federal Gun Control Act was passed in 1968, around which time too state and local governments passed hundreds of additional gun control laws.
- According to the *Statistical Abstract of the United States* there was a 20 percent decline in killings provoked in the course of arguments between 1980 and 1992, the opposite of what the instrumentality theory predicts.
- The suicide rate in the United States is not correlated at all with the availability of firearms, contrary to one of the main predictions of the instrumentality theory.
- There is considerable evidence, gathered by Professor John Lott of the University of Chicago Law School, that states that have loosened their "concealed carry" laws with regard to handguns have experienced *declining* firearm violence and violent crime rates, also contrary to the instru-

mentality theory. For example, Florida liberalized its concealed-carry law in 1988, when it had one of the nation's highest murder rates. The state's murder rate has fallen in every year since the law was changed. In 1988 Florida's homicide rate was 37 percent above the national average; today it is 3 percent *below* the national average. The first reaction of the public health "establishment" was not to debate Professor Lott, but to insinuate that he was an intellectual prostitute, "paid off" by the conservative Olin Foundation, which funded his fellowship at the University of Chicago. (In reality, the Olin money goes directly to the law school, and hundreds of applicants compete for the prestigious fellowship. Professor Lott is one of the most prolific scholars in the economics profession, which is why he was awarded the fellowship).[29]

Like religious zealots, the CDC-funded gun control researchers are absolutists in their beliefs. They know of the research showing that there are millions of defensive uses of firearms each year, which implies that the "trade-off" one would be compelled to accept if guns were completely banned would likely be millions of additional injuries and deaths of innocent people at the hands of criminals. But we should not be allowed to make this trade-off for ourselves, the gun control advocates argue, for they are RIGHT.

A recent example of this support for governmental compulsion, no matter how counterproductive, is the political push to require firearms manufacturers to put "childproof gun locks" on their products. As of this writing, some state legislatures have enacted such legislation and the federal government was debating it.

Assuming that it is technologically feasible to render firearms "childproof," even this kind of legislation eliminates a degree of freedom of choice and will inevitably cause more deaths from firearms. The reason is that a locked, unloaded gun provides much less protection from intruders. Thus, requiring gun locks will increase deaths resulting from crime.[30]

## Disregarding Constitutional Liberties

The CDC's funding of gun control "studies" under the assumption that guns are a "virus" and that gun ownership is a "disease" is absurd, especially coming from an organization comprised supposedly of medical professionals. Gun ownership usually does not lead to violence, and much violence occurs without the appearance of a gun. Depicting gun ownership as a "disease"— even when dressed up in a pseudo-scientific sounding, "peer-reviewed" public health "journal"— is simply intellectually dishonest.

Of course, some of the CDC-funded "research" is not research at all, but political training in "media advocacy," that is, lobbying. Thus, we have the spectacle of taxpayers' dollars being used to finance political campaigns to undermine a constitutionally protected freedom. If gun control advocates at the CDC want to abolish the Second Amendment to the U.S. Constitution, they should do so by trying to amend the Constitution, not through legislation based on politically contrived and methodologically flawed "studies."

The public health profession is heavily involved in a political crusade to invent new "rights" (through legislation and regulation) that are not mentioned in the Constitution, such as the alleged "right" to get other taxpayers to pay for one's health care bills, while undermining various rights that actually are in the Constitution, such as the Second Amendment's right to bear arms. This is apparently what authors Lawrence Wallack and Lori Dorfman, mentioned at the outset of this chapter, meant when, in a publication widely distributed to CDC employees, they urged public health professionals to "rethink the foundation of basic values on which society is based."[31]

When the neurosurgeon Faria was fired for publishing an exchange of views on gun control, the *Atlanta Journal and Constitution* ridiculed him in an editorial for harboring the misguided belief that the Constitution actually permitted gun ownership. The paper called the idea that "the Second Amendment was plainly intended to guarantee the right of individuals to own guns" a "howler." This intolerance reflects the attitude taken by the CDC and its well-paid researchers who were intended to be the direct beneficiaries of the Atlanta paper's editorial. But there are legal scholars who, even though they personally oppose gun ownership, have acknowledged that the Second Amendment does indeed protect the right to bear arms. Among the most prominent is Sanford Levinson, a professor of law at the University of Texas, author of the most widely used law school text on the Constitution, *Processes of Constitutional Decision Making*, and a frequent participant in ACLU litigation.

In a *Yale Law Journal* article entitled "The Embarrassing Second Amendment" Professor Levinson admits that the Second Amendment protects the right to bear arms and admonishes his fellow firearm prohibitionists "who want to square their policy preferences with the Constitution" to "squarely face the need to deconstitutionalize the subject by repealing the embarrassing amendment."[32] In other words, quit trying to subvert the Second Amendment through unconstitutional legislation and regulation — amend the Constitution instead.

Another particularly candid legal scholar is Professor Akhil Amar who, also writing in the *Yale Law Journal*, clearly explained why the Second Amendment gives *the people*, not the states or the national guard, the right to bear arms, as gun control advocates often assert. "When the Constitution means 'states' it says so.... The ultimate right to keep and bear arms belongs to the people, not the states."[33]

In her 1994 book, *To Keep and Bear Arms: The Origins of an Anglo-American Right*, published by Harvard University Press, Professor Joyce Malcolm concurs that the Second Amendment was intended to guarantee the individual's right to self-defense and self-preservation, and to be part of a voluntary, citizen militia whose purpose was to thwart unconstitutional governmental power. "The argument that today's National Guardsmen, members of a select militia, would constitute the only persons entitled to keep and bear arms has no historical foundation."[34]

This is not meant to be a comprehensive review of the Second Amendment literature. The point is to show that there is a solid scholarly foundation for the belief that the Second Amendment guarantees the right of individuals to own firearms. Those who ridicule that idea do so out of ignorance, arrogance, elitism, and intolerance of opposing viewpoints.

Indeed, when one closely examines the case for gun control, it is hard to find *any* evidence that it could in any way improve public health. After all, Washington, D.C. has had the strictest gun control laws in the nation since 1976, and it is still referred to as the "murder capital" of the United States. If gun control worked, it should work in Washington, D.C. Crime has become so out of control in the nation's capital that the police have begun training citizens in the safe use of shotguns. (It has been illegal to own a handgun there since 1976.) So, the strictest gun control laws in the nation have not deterred violent criminals, who don't pay attention to such laws, while law-abiding citizens remain largely defenseless. Yet the CDC continues to use tax dollars to fund seminars and newsletters on how to adopt Washington, D.C.-style gun control legislation in more American cities. Surely, there are more direct ways to improve public health in America — the ostensible purpose of the CDC.

# 6

# Can Tax-Funded Lobbying Cure Disease?

> *"Call it 'policy advocacy,' 'media advocacy,' 'changing the social environment;' if it looks like lobbying, talks like lobbying, sounds like lobbying — it's lobbying! And taxpayers don't want their tax dollars paying bureaucrats to lobby cities and states."*
> —*The Advocacy Institute*[1]

For fifty years the federal government's Centers for Disease Control (CDC) has been concerned with curing disease through research, public education, and inoculation. But recently the CDC has been shifting its focus from the practice of medicine and medical research to politics. The agency now spends tens of millions of taxpayers' dollars annually *to train lobbyists* on how to get gun control laws enacted, as seen in the last chapter, how to ban smoking or tobacco advertising, and on other politically correct causes.

It is illegal to use tax dollars for partisan politics, so there are serious concerns about the CDC's political initiatives. This chapter examines a major national program funded by the CDC that spent $85 million in tax dollars in 1993 alone to initiate a program in 32 states and the District of Columbia to train lobbyists and build political coalitions that will advocate banning tobacco products.

No one today denies the health hazards of smoking; the issue is not whether smoking is healthy; it is not. Rather, the issue is whether or not prohibition is wise public policy and, more importantly, whether or not tax dollars ought to be used to promote it.

Once tax dollars are used to prohibit one kind of politically incorrect consumption behavior, there is in principle no end to it. Today, smoking happens to be the most politically incorrect behavior, but the consumption of fast foods, alcohol, red meat, and myriad other products arguably posing some degree of detriment to the public's health have already been attacked by various public health groups. In light of this, a look at the CDC's approach to smoking control provides some

65

insight into how the "new public health" process works and how various groups gain control of taxpayer's public health money.

## The CDC's IMPACT Grant Program

In 1993 the CDC's Office on Smoking and Health awarded $85 million to 32 state health departments as part of its "National Tobacco Prevention and Control Program," which the agency labels Initiatives to Mobilize for the Prevention And Control of Tobacco Use (IMPACT).[2] The grants to state health departments are renewable for up to five years.

At first blush there does not seem to be anything objectionable to state health departments helping people to quit smoking or discouraging them — especially children — from starting to smoke in the first place. But the primary emphasis of the program is not medical treatment or education but politics. The essential purpose of the grants is to mobilize a "comprehensive and coordinated nationwide effort" to enact prohibitionist legislation with "local, state, and regional initiatives."[3]

Florida — essentially a model for what the CDC hopes to achieve in the other thirty-one states and the District of Columbia — has received significant funding (approximately $250,000 per year since 1993) from the CDC's IMPACT program and will be the focus of this inquiry.

The grants fall into two categories: "planning awards" for states that have not yet established a political coalition, and "core awards" to assist states that have already established the political infrastructure for such a coalition. The targeted states are as listed in table 6.1.

### TABLE 6.1

#### States Targeted for CDC IMPACT Grants

| Planning Award States | Core Award States |
|---|---|
| Alabama, Arizona, Arkansas, Connecticut Delaware, Georgia, Kentucky, Mississippi, Nevada, Oregon, S. Dakota, Tennessee, Wyoming, Vermont | Alaska, District of Columbia, Florida, Hawaii, Idaho, Illinois, Iowa, Kansas, Louisiana, Maryland, Montana, Nebraska, New Hampshire, N. Dakota, Ohio, Oklahoma, Pennsylvania, Texas, Utah |

Source: U.S. Department of Health and Human Services, Centers for Disease Control, "National Tobacco Prevention and Control Program," 1994.

In its initial 1993 grant proposal to the CDC, the Florida Department of Health and Rehabilitative Services (FDHRS) "project director," Joyner Sims, explained that the money would be spent mobilizing a "Tobacco Free Florida Coalition."[4] At the time, this political coalition was known as "The American Cancer Society's Lung Cancer Task Force," indicating that the apparent purpose of the grant was to use taxpayers' dollars to fund this ACS program. The grant paid the salary of the person who is the "Tobacco Free Florida Coalition Coordinator," a position that "is located at the American Cancer Society (ACS) in Tampa, Florida," according to the grant contract.[5]

In its application to the CDC the FDHRS listed a need to fill certain political "gaps" in the state, including:

- Lack of a comprehensive statewide political coalition;
- Limited funding for local political coalition building;
- "Undirected" local political coalitions that are in need of direction in the area of "cultural diversity";
- Lack of adequate staff at the state government level to help build these political coalitions.[6]

Among the policies the FDHRS promised to lobby for with federal tax dollars are:

- Local ordinances that would ban smoking in the workplace;
- "Educational campaigns for lawmakers";
- Cigarette vending machine bans;
- Tobacco products advertising restrictions;
- Tobacco excise tax increases, with some of the revenues earmarked for members of the Tobacco Free Florida Coalition;
- Banning promotional giveaways of tobacco products;
- Banning the sale of cigarettes by pharmacies; and
- Raising the legal smoking age to twenty-one.[7]

In addition to paying at least part of the salaries of Florida Health Department employees, ACS staff, and newly hired political activists and consultants, the grant covers "travel expenses for coalition members to attend quarterly meetings," "meeting room costs," the printing of a semi-annual coalition newsletter, and "mini-grants" to local political coalitions throughout the state.

The exact role of the tax-funded Tobacco Free Florida Coalition is also described in the proposal:

- "Provide advocacy" for "tobacco prevention and control legislation" and "develop new legislation specifically targeting restrictions on outdoor advertising";
- Develop a "formal network contact information collection and dissemination framework" for the coalition;

- Provide all coalition members and network contacts with a listing of data-bases and resources;
- Develop a political "training and technical assistance plan" to provide "co-ordinated support" for lobbyists;
- Fund travel of coalition members to political training conferences to attain "more specialized" lobbying and advocacy skills; and
- Develop "a linkage with the Florida Association of Broadcasters."

Taxpayers' funds also helped finance the coalition's participation in SCARCNet, an on-line communication network used by anti-smoking political activists that "allows state officials to coordinate with CDC officials in countering major tobacco industry announcements."[8]

The role of the major health charities — the ACS, American Heart Association (AHA), and American Lung Association (ALA) — and the political nature of the IMPACT grant program — can be seen in the grant application's table listing the personnel of the coalition. What the table shows is that the health charities are all effectively receiving tax-payers' dollars as members of this coalition, and that what they are engaged in is arguably illegal, tax-funded political advocacy. Some of the members of the coalition are listed in table 6.2, with their roles in the coalition as described by the FDHRS grant application.

**TABLE 6.2**

**Members of the Tobacco Free Florida Coalition**

| Coalition Member | Organization Represented | Role in the Coalition |
| --- | --- | --- |
| Don Webster | American Cancer Society | Legislation expertise, grass roots mobilization |
| John J. Brennan | American Heart Association | Grass roots mobilization |
| Sandra Kessler | American Lung Association | Grass roots mobilization |
| Dennis Valera | American Cancer Society | Coalition builder |
| Frederick Schild | Florida Medical Association | Lobbying assistance |
| Beatrice Braun | American Assoc. of Retired Persons | Advocacy Services |
| Higuel DeGrandy | Florida Hispanic Legislative Caucus | Legislative assistance |
| George Albright | State Legislator | Policymaking |
| Beth Labasky | Registered Lobbyist | Legislative expert |
| Marcia Nenno | American Cancer Society | Coalition building |

*Source*: Florida Department of Health and Rehabilitative Services, Grant Proposal to Centers for Disease Control, 1993, obtained through Freedom of Information Act request.

There are also medical professionals on the list of coalition members, but in virtually every instance their role is listed as a liaison with fellow professionals, that is, as a political operative, not as a medical professional, per se.

## The Role of the Robert Wood Johnson Foundation

A key player in the politicization of public health is the Robert Wood Johnson Foundation (RWJF). In Florida and in twenty other states, RWJF is supplementing taxpayer funding by the CDC with its "Smokeless States" grant program. According to a foundation brochure describing the program, the foundation "will make new grants to up to 21 statewide coalitions working in partnership with community groups."[9] RWJF hopes that its grants will "strengthen state-wide coalitions" and plans to spend $20 million in the next four years on the program. The funds will be devoted to "mobilizing state-wide coalitions" as well as waging public education campaigns about smoking.

The involvement of the RWJF in such a politicized enterprise shouldn't be a surprise. Located in Princeton, New Jersey, it was founded in 1972 and is the largest private foundation in the U.S. devoted exclusively to health care issues. Its assets approach $4 billion and its major health policy initiatives are almost exclusively aimed at massively increasing the amount of government intervention in health care.[10]

Lawsuits against Hillary Clinton's secret health care task force revealed that the RWJF had a profound influence on the construction of the Clinton administration's attempt at a governmental takeover of the entire private health care system in 1993 and 1994.

Under its "State Initiatives in Health Care Reform" program, RWJF has put millions of dollars behind political lobbying efforts to pass health care reform laws in individual states that possess many of the features of the failed Clinton health plan, such as price controls, mandated managed care, "community rating" of health insurance, and regulation of health care markets. Florida, Minnesota, and Washington have passed legislation favored by the RWJF. Such laws apparently "allow state officials to circumvent a U.S. Congress that is unwilling to do what the [Clinton] administration and RWJF know is best."[11]

In keeping with the political focus of the Tobacco Free Florida Coalition, the foundation is supporting political efforts to: (a) increase state tobacco excise taxes and earmarking some of the revenue to the health charities and other members of its coalitions; (b) promote local ordinances that ban smoking; (c) ban smoking in the workplace; (d) reduce youth access to tobacco products; and (e) change Medicaid so that "tobacco cessation services," provided by the health charities, among others, are covered.

To qualify for the RWJF grants, as Florida has, one must demonstrate the existence of a "strong, broad-based state-wide coalition," a "state government commitment to the effort including support from the governor, key legislators, and other public officials," and "recent or proposed local and state policy and financing changes" designed to achieve tobacco prohibition.[12] And prohibition is what RWJF and the health charities are advocating, despite their occasional protests that they are not "prohibitionists." How else, after all, could one interpret the phrase, "Smokeless States"?

In Florida, RWJF provides in-kind as well as financial support: "The Robert Wood Johnson Foundation Advocacy Coordinators are assisting the [CDC] funded tobacco coalitions" with their political activities, notes a 1996 FDHRS "progress report" to the CDC. Among other things, these "advocacy coordinators" are organizing media campaigns, taking opinion polls, and training people in political advocacy. The RWJF grant is also being used in Florida to bring in "nationally recognized experts in the tobacco control movement." These experts are likely from the Washington, D.C.-based Advocacy Institute, a liberal activist group directed by former Carter administration official Michael Pertschuk.

All these efforts by RWJF are in keeping with its past record of trying to "solve" public health problems with more government bureaucracy, more regulation, and more taxes.

## Using Children as Political Pawns

For decades the political left has used children as an excuse to enact public policies which primarily affect adults. The Children's Defense Fund, for example, spends most of its resources lobbying for an expanded welfare state. Its name is very useful politically; it can accuse critics of the failed welfare state programs as being "anti-children."

The CDC and RWJF have adopted this strategy by including programs aimed at children, although most of the policy recommendations they make, such as higher excise taxes, would affect everyone. In Florida and in other IMPACT states, school children are encouraged (and sometimes paid) to join the Student Coalition Against Tobacco (SCAT) and to help "launch a SCAT campaign."[13] SCAT organizes myriad activities for students, and all of them are "considered youth political advocacy, which is at the very base of the Student Coalition Against Tobacco."[14]

The ACS, AHA, and ALA oversee SCAT activities and teach children to demonize their political opponents. Join SCAT, children are told, and begin "counteracting immoral tobacco industry tactics."[15]

There is nothing wrong with schoolchildren advising their friends to avoid taking up smoking. Junior high and high school students are paid by SCAT to conduct private sting operations directed at convenience stores. These operations involve "sending minors out into the community in an attempt to purchase cigarettes either over the counter in retail outlets or from vending machines located in stores, restaurants, bars or other locations."[16] Such practices have been criticized by California law enforcement officials as "vigilantism," but are nevertheless an integral part of the CDC's national coalition-building campaign.

Much of the information given to SCAT recruits by the health charities is questionable. For example, an instructional guide advises children to "make the public aware that young people are being attacked by toxins whenever we eat in a restaurant, play pool or bowl, or attend school."[17] But, as yet, there is no solid evidence that second-hand smoke is as hazardous as such a statement implies it is — if, indeed, it poses any significant risk at all. Students who do not understand this, however, are only needlessly frightened by such hysteria.

### Political "Progress"

The CDC requires its thirty-two state grantees to issue "progress reports" annually. Florida's reports for 1993-95 show that, although some of the funds are spent on public education programs, the lion's share goes toward tax-funded politics and are therefore probably illegally spent. From September 1993 to May 1994 the FDHRS boasted of lobbying for a $1 increase in the state's tobacco products tax, working closely with AHA lobbyist Scott Ballin. Their effort was unsuccessful.

Also, the sting operations conducted by "underage operatives who are observed by a special enforcement agent" resulted in hundreds of convenience store clerks being entrapped and cited; dozens of businesses having "administrative actions" taken against their business licenses; and a "total of $136,000 in fees were collected for the Department of Education."[18]

One might ask, however, whether or not there isn't something unsavory about Florida Department of Education bureaucrats paying other peoples' children to conduct vigilante-style sting operations that entrap fellow citizens just to enlarge the bureaucrats' budgets. In light of the crisis in American primary and secondary education and the failures of so many public schools to teach children how to read, write, and communicate, it hardly seems appropriate for a state Department of Education to use children as political pawns in budget games.

Furthermore, with all the serious crime problems, one has to wonder about the propriety of tying up law enforcement resources by arresting convenience store clerks for selling cigarettes to 17 1/2-year-olds. Does this really advance the cause of public health?

If teenagers want to smoke they will obtain cigarettes somehow. Arresting even hundreds of convenience store clerks in Florida will not deter teenage smoking; it will only garner temporary headlines for the Tobacco Free Florida Coalition. The overall health of Florida's teenagers will not be improved, but the health of people who typically staff the cash registers at convenience stores may be harmed if they lose their jobs and suffer declines in their incomes.

Perhaps the most important political "progress" reported to the CDC is that the coalition helped lobby for a new law, SB 2110, enacted on May 25, 1994, that allowed the state to sue the tobacco industry to recover health care costs from tobacco-related illnesses incurred by Medicaid recipients. Florida argued that tobacco companies should be liable for the negative health effects of their product even if smokers know full well that smoking increases health risks. If this argument is accepted by the courts, it is hard to imagine that plaintiffs' lawyers will not file similar class action lawsuits against the alcoholic beverage industry, the fast food business, and other industries.

Nevertheless, the National Cancer Institute (NCI) is teaming up with the CDC to achieve just such an outcome. According to NCI grant # CA-94-15, obtained through a Freedom of Information Act request, Northeastern University Law School in Boston received $1,119,678 in 1995 for a four-year legal research project that will "produce policy papers" on "states' ability to sue tobacco companies for the medical expenditures caused by tobacco-related diseases" and paid from Medicaid. The grantees — law professors and their students at the university — will also research "the optimal design and constitutional validity of state legislation that would strengthen legal procedures for obtaining such reimbursement of health care costs from the tobacco industry." Additional government funding for the project was provided by the Massachusetts Department of Public Health ($324,500 annually) and the Americans With Disabilities Act ($284,804). To be sure, the mega-millionaire plaintiffs lawyers who have taken such cases on behalf of the states, such as Baltimore Orioles owner Peter Angelos in the case of Maryland, could well afford their own legal research, especially since they stand to earn hundreds of millions of dollars in contingency fees. But such is the nature of public health spending these days.

Finally, another piece of "progress" reported to CDC is that FDHRS recruited an attorney to help employees harass their employers who fail to enact anti-smoking policies along the lines suggested by the state coalition: The coalition will use federal tax dollars to "actively support employee litigation against employers who fail to implement meaningful smoking policies."[19]

### Resurrecting Alcohol Prohibition

The Robert Wood Johnson Foundation has also announced a new four-year, $10.2 million grant program that follows the exact same format as its "Tobacco Free States" grant program. The new program will fund statewide political coalitions as well as local coalitions with the objective of encouraging alcohol prohibition. Like the anti-smoking programs there is a lot of rhetoric about children. Indeed, the name of the new program is "Reducing Underage Drinking Through Community and State Coalitions."[20] But the specific public policies that are highlighted in the brochure announcing the new program are ones that would affect *everyone* — underage as well as legal drinkers.

For example, among government interventions "shown to be effective" are "restrictions on the distribution of alcohol" through state government monopoly liquor stores, regulatory limits on "outlet density," and the elimination of advertising. State liquor stores, because they are monopolies, charge higher prices than private, competitive liquor stores do, so that all adult purchasers of liquor would be made worse off. Limits on "outlet density," moreover, would probably only cause people to drive further away from home in order to drink, thus, perversely, causing traffic hazards. And by restricting or limiting advertising, any remaining price competition in the industry will be weakened, which will also lead to higher liquor prices.

Another "effective" intervention, according to RWJF, is "increases in taxes and the relative price of alcoholic beverages."[21] Again, this is all promoted in the name of children, but the above-mentioned laws and regulations apply to adults, not sales to minors, which are already illegal. There is no mention at all in the RWJF literature about *parental responsibility* in teaching children not to abuse liquor; to RWJF, apparently, all such responsibility should rest in the hands of the state.

In the very last paragraph of its grant announcement RWJF oddly states that "grant funds may not be used ... for lobbying or otherwise attempting to influence legislation." Yet the entire thrust of the program is precisely to fund statewide coalitions *of lobbyists* to try to enact the above-mentioned prohibitionist policies. Grantees are "expected to mobilize existing or new statewide or local coalitions" to enact higher alcohol excise taxes and other legislated restrictions on alcohol consumption. Among the "selection criteria" for the grants is the "*political feasibility*" of the state's project (emphasis added).

These prohibitionist policies are "seen as the most successful approaches," according to the RWJF brochure, which is why it is allocating $10.2 million to finance *lobbying* campaigns in at least twelve states initially.

## Conclusions

It is illegal to spend tax funds on partisan political activity, yet the CDC is doing exactly that by allocating hundreds of millions of tax dollars for political coalition building. These sums are comparable to the amounts spent on congressional campaigns in a given year.

The role of the Robert Wood Johnson Foundation is also interesting in this regard. Individuals and organizations that make campaign contributions cannot deduct the contributions from their taxes. But RWJF is a tax-exempt foundation that is spending millions of dollars constructing the "political infrastructure" for various prohibitionist political movements in dozens of states. This, too, is of questionable legality.

Financial self-interest is also at play. Consider the role of the major health charities — the ACS, AHA, and ALA — in tax-funded politics by the CDC. As documented, the health charities are often recipients of some of the funds, and the political coalitions they are building with the funds lobby state legislatures to *require* various educational programs for both adults and children that would be administered by none other than the health charities.[22]

Since general economic ignorance is also a threat to the nation's "health," this would be akin to the authors' professional organization — the American Economic Association — using tax dollars to lobby for laws that *required* states to pay economics professors to provide lectures to various members of the public, whether the public wanted them or not. Such a scheme would be "rationalized" with "public interest" rhetoric, but it would in reality be an attempt by economists to plunder the taxpayers for their own benefit.

By shifting its focus from health research, education, and disease inoculation to political campaigns for politically correct behavior, the CDC has not only crossed the line into legally questionable activities, but has been wasting scarce public health resources.

# 7

# Nothing But Politics

*"We need your help. Drop everything and write your congressman."*
—The Nation's Health, *"Action Alert"*

If one wonders how "public health" has drifted so far from its moorings in traditional public health practices, look no further than the principal group representing the public health establishment for the answer.

As a 501(c)(3) nonprofit organization, the American Public Health Association (APHA) is limited in the amount of lobbying activities in which it may legally engage. In the parlance of the IRS, a 501(c)(4) "nonprofit" organization is one that can legally lobby with all its resources. Many of the former type of nonprofit organizations that engage in educational or charitable endeavors also create the latter type of organization for their lobbying efforts.

Despite its tax classification and its self-description as a "nongovernmental professional society," reading the association's flagship monthly publication, *The Nation's Health*, gives one the clear impression that the association is primarily a lobbying organization and only secondarily an association for health professionals. Through its monthly publication the association issues frequent "Action Alerts" to its members with such messages as "We need your help. Your Senator is an influential member of the Senate Commerce committee.... Please contact your senator and urge him to co-sponsor and support this crucial legislation."[1] The association "has continued to maintain a strong presence on Capital Hill," says one membership renewal letter which also boasts of how politically active the association has been: Attendees at the 1993 annual meeting "wrote 2,576 letters to Congress on computer terminals provided by APHA."[2] Of course, since the APHA receives federal funds (and it is illegal to use federal funds for partisan political purposes), all this politicking raises further questions regarding legality, as well as propriety.

The underlying premise of the APHA's political activities, as noted earlier, is that "organizing" and political "activism" are routes to improved public health. But many of the policies advocated by the public health establishment are clearly of questionable value to public health. Many others seem to have little or no relation at all to it; they simply reflect the political proclivities of the establishment's leadership. This political mind-set favors bigger government, more bureaucracy, more taxes, and more regulation.

## Can Politics Cure Disease?

As an international organization that claims over 50,000 members worldwide one would expect at least some ideological diversity on some issues, but there is none. The professional association that purportedly represents the views of the public health profession is uniformly on the left of the political spectrum on every issue, from international family planning to the balanced budget, to immigration policy.

## Maximum Abortion

The APHA's lobbyists support government-funded abortion and abortion training, having lobbied for federal funding of international "family planning" activities and for increased funding to medical schools to train abortion doctors. Without getting into the abortion issue, it is interesting to note that legal abortion procedures themselves have caused serious health problems — and even deaths — with thousands of women, yet one cannot find any mention of concern about *this* public health issue in any of the APHA's literature. It is routinely assumed that legal abortions are "safe" and that making it illegal will cause injury and death. The APHA would mention this if its objective were purely the pursuit of better public health and not to push a social and political agenda.

The APHA, which purportedly represents *all* public health professionals, even comes down hard on one side of the extraordinarily divisive issue of partial birth abortion — a procedure even abortion supporters, such as former U.S. Senator Daniel Patrick Moynihan (D-N.Y.), oppose as being "too close to infanticide." At the same time, the APHA supports increases in federal funding of "early-stage embryo research" — medical research that makes use of the corpses of aborted babies.[3] The association's lobbyists have also opposed a bill that would have required government-funded family planning clinics, such as Planned Parenthood, to notify the parents of minors seeking abortions. The association does not want parental involvement in teenage abortion decisions because that will "result in unwanted teen pregnancies."[4]

## Denial of Health Care Choice

The public health establishment may be "pro-choice" on abortion, but is adamantly opposed to choice when it comes to health care spending. For example, the APHA lobbyists also supported an "effort to eliminate the provisions for medical savings accounts" from a Senate bill. Medical Savings Accounts are a health-insurance financing vehicle intended to expand the degree of consumer choice and price competition in the purchase of medical care. Once widely established, these accounts would both increase consumer sovereignty in a market dominated by insurer and HMO decision making and reduce health-cost inflation, which stems from the distorted market incentives created by the third-party payment dominance of insurers, HMOs, and the government in health care spending. Better, in short, to give consumers more health care buying power, while maintaining insurance for catastrophically costly medical care.

The idea is fairly straightforward. If employers currently spend, say, $5,000 per year per employee on health insurance, at present all that money goes to the health insurer or HMO. If no health care is sought over the year, all that money stays with these third-party payers, which just encourages consumers, in a sense, to get their money's worth by using available health care as much as possible. (It is virtually free for the consumer at the point of consumption after all.) This is why there is price inflation and the resulting clamp down on demand through "gate keepers," managed care, care denial, and the like. So, rather than giving the entire $5,000 to insurers, under a Medical Savings Account, the $5,000 would become the property of the employee and placed into a tax-exempt savings account. The employee then would be required to purchase a less-expensive, high-deductible ($2,000 or $3,000) health insurance policy. This would cover major medical expenses, while the remaining $3,000 or so could be used towards the deductible over the year. Any money remaining at the end of the year — and for many people in any given year there would be some — remains in the account to accumulate tax free, much like an Individual Retirement Account. Once employees realize that it is *their* money, they are bound to spend it as wisely as they can, so they can build their accounts for future health spending, retirement, emergencies, a source of income when between jobs, and so on.

Several private companies, such as the Golden Rule Insurance Company in Indianapolis, Indiana, and *Forbes* magazine have adopted medical savings accounts for their own employees and have found that their health care costs have dropped while the degree of employee satisfaction with their health care coverage has improved. Expanding this concept to more employees and to Medicare recipients — as is happening now in the United States — would very likely have the same effect, since freedom of consumer choice and competition always lead to better products and services at lower costs.

But an expanded degree of consumer choice and competition is exactly the opposite of what the public health establishment wants. The public health establishment is committed to government control of health care, which means a health care system run as a government monopoly, which means no consumer control over spending and certainly no consumer incentive to spend wisely and save for future benefit. Medical savings accounts, *The Nation's Health* explained, are unacceptable because by giving Americans greater freedom of choice over their own health care choices they constitute "obstacles to universal coverage."[5]

## Welfare as the Magic Cure-All

· APHA lobbyists vigorously supported an expansion of the American welfare system, believing that being on welfare is conducive to improved public health. Accordingly, APHA lobbyists "participated in several coalitions" and distributed a position paper by the association's president, E. Richard Brown, on the floor of the U.S. Senate that opposed placing restrictions on the ability of illegal immigrants to receive welfare benefits, including Medicaid.

Similarly, efforts to devolve welfare control to the states has been steadfastly opposed. Several bills in the 104th Congress would have allowed states to set their own eligibility standards for Medicaid. These bills were all opposed by APHA lobbyists, as were efforts to include food stamps in block grants to the states from the federal government.

However, these efforts were to no avail: Congress and the president enacted a welfare reform bill in 1996 that begins phasing out welfare spending by ending the federal guarantee of welfare benefits, giving states greater latitude in administering welfare programs, limiting recipients to five years on the dole, and requiring able-bodied welfare recipients to find work within a prescribed time period. Yet, the APHA continues to oppose this reform by "working with coalition partners concerned about children."

Expanding the welfare state "for the children" is an appealing plea to many Americans, but there is voluminous evidence that the welfare state itself has been very harmful to children. One of the principal claims of the proponents of higher welfare spending, for example, is that children in low-income families with higher welfare payments (which vary considerably by state) will have improved cognitive ability because of better nutrition, housing, and so on. But economists June O'Neill, former director of the Congressional Budget Office, and Anne Hill of Queens College reported in the peer-reviewed *Journal of Human Resources* that "the IQs of long-term welfare-dependent children in low-benefit states were not appreciably different from those in high-benefit states."[6]

Moreover, welfare itself had negative effects. Hill and O'Neill also found that the longer a child's family stays on welfare the *lower* his or her IQ tends to be. These authors found that it is not poverty, per se, that is the problem, but being on welfare. Examining a sample of five-year-olds, the authors concluded that children who had spent at least two months of each year since birth on Aid to Families with Dependent Children (AFDC) had cognitive abilities 20 percent below those who had received no welfare, even after controlling for family income, race, parental IQ, and other variables.

Another study by University of Michigan researchers found that being on welfare has a powerful negative impact on the earning ability of young boys.[7] The study compared families whose average non-welfare incomes were identical and determined that each extra dollar in welfare income negatively affected the development of young boys within the family and that every $1,000 in annual welfare income reduced the boys' future earnings by as much as 10 percent.

Other studies have found that young women raised in families dependent on welfare are two to three times more likely to drop out, and fail to graduate from high school, than are young women of similar race and socioeconomic backgrounds who are not raised on welfare.[8] Single mothers raised as children in families receiving welfare also tend to remain on welfare longer as adult parents than do single mothers who were not raised on welfare, even after controlling for other socioeconomic variables.[9]

It has also been well established by social science research that welfare promotes illegitimacy. The explanation for this phenomenon is what economists call the moral hazard problem. Currently, a single mother with two children is eligible to receive up to $15,000 annually (depending on her state of residence) in welfare payments. She is only eligible for the funds, however, as long as she does not marry an employed man. Welfare thus makes marriage economically irrational, and has made it easier to raise a child without either the father or mother holding a job or, indeed, without the father even being present. Herein lies the "moral hazard": In attempting to help unwed mothers, welfare policy has created more unwed mothers by giving fathers an "excuse" to become derelict in the responsibilities they have for their offspring. (This is not true of everyone, of course, but it is true for a sizable number of men).

Research by Hill and O'Neill also indicates that, after controlling for such variables as income, parental education, and urban and neighborhood setting, a 50 percent increase in the monthly value of AFDC and food stamp benefits leads to a 43 percent increase in the number of out-of-wedlock births.[10] Numerous other studies provide additional evidence of the positive correlation between welfare payments and illegitimacy, as shown in table 7.1.

There have been a few studies that show no statistically significant relationship between welfare payments and illegitimacy, but none has ever found welfare to have a positive effect on reducing illegitimacy and promoting marriage.[11]

From the perspective of public health, these research results should be most alarming. Indeed, they should cause one to question the public health establishment's strong endorsement of an ever-bigger welfare state. There is growing evidence that children born out of wedlock have a much higher probability of suffering from retarded cognitive development,[12] lower educational achievement and job attainment,[13] increased behavioral and emotional problems, and retarded social development.[14] Such children are more likely to engage in early sexual activity, have children out of wedlock, end up on welfare as adults, and engage in criminal activity. A major 1988 study found that the failure to form and maintain intact families explains much of the incidence of high teenage crime rates within neighborhoods populated by all different races, and that illegitimacy, not poverty, explains the incidence of teenage crime in the neighborhoods studied.[15] Meanwhile, the APHA lobbies on.

## TABLE 7.1

### Selected Research on Welfare and Illegitimacy

| Authors/Study | Results |
| --- | --- |
| M. Bernstam, "Malthus and the Evolution of the Welfare State," Hoover Institution, Working Paper E-88-41,42, 1988 | 10% increase in welfare leads to 6% increase in illegitimacy |
| M.A.Fossett and K.J. Kiecolt, "Mate Availability and Family Structure Among African Americans in U.S. Metropolitan Areas," *Journal of Marriage and Family*, vol. 55, May 1993 | $100 monthly increase in AFDC payments leads to 15% drop in births within wedlock |
| C.R. Winegarden, "AFDC and Illegitimacy Ratios: A Vector-Autoregressive Model," *Applied Economics*, vol. 20, 1988 | Half the increase in black illegitimacy rates in recent decades caused by welfare |
| S. Lundberg and R. Plotnick, "Adolescent Premarital Child Bearing," Univ. of Washington, Institute for Economic Research, 1990 | $200 increase in monthly welfare payment leads to 150% increase in teen illegitimate birth rate |
| M. Ozawa, "Welfare Policies and Illegitimate Birth Rates Among Adolescents," *National Work Research and Abstracts*, vol. 14, 1989 | $100 per month increase in AFDC payments leads to 30% increase in teenage illegitimate births |
| M. Rosenzweig, "Welfare, Marital Prospects and Nonmarital Childbearing," National Academy of Sciences, December 1995 | $140 per month reduction in AFDC payments leads to 40% drop in teenage out-of-wedlock births |
| C. An, R. Haveman, B. Wolfe, "Teen Out-of-Wedlock Births and Welfare Receipt," *Review of Economics and Statistics*, vol. 75, May 1993 | 20% increase in welfare benefit levels leads to 16% more illegitimate births |
| C. Murray, "Welfare and the Family: The U.S. Experience," *Journal of Labor Economics*, vol. 11, 1993 | Higher welfare causes higher illegitimacy |
| P. Schultz, "Marital Status and Fertility in the United States," *Journal of Human Resources*, vol. 29, Spring 1994 | Higher welfare benefits reduce marriage rates |
| S. South and K. Lloyd, "Marriage Markets and Fertility in the U.S.," *Demography*, vol. 29, May 1992 | Positive relationship between welfare payments and percentage of births that are out of wedlock |
| P. Robins and P. Fronton, "Welfare Benefits and Family Size Decisions of Never-Married Women, "Institute for Research on Poverty Discussion Paper # DP 1022-93, Univ. of Wisconsin, 1993 | Higher welfare benefits lead to more births among never-married women |

## In the Name of Environmentalism

In 1996 the APHA joined a coalition of environmental organizations that was formed to lobby for the EPA's proposed new air-quality standards. As usual, the increased regulation was sold in the name of "the children." "When it comes to protecting our kids, I won't be swayed," pronounced an indignant EPA administrator Carol Browner.[16] Whatever the merits of the clean air initiatives, they were known to be costly, extremely costly, with only small anticipated benefit.

For example, estimates for tightening smog-control standards proposed by the EPA in 1996 would have run between $2.5 billion and $7 billion annually, or more, depending on who made the estimate. Benefits, in terms of reduced health care costs, ranged from around $33 million to just over $1 billion. But the science behind these benefit estimates was questioned, even by the EPA's own scientific advisory panel.[17] To put the benefits in more perspective, consider that tightening the ozone standard in the New York City area would cut asthma hospital admissions by an estimated 0.5 percent — or about 100 out of 28,000.[18]

In some instances the EPA/APHA regulatory policy actually threatens to harm hundreds, if not thousands, of children, and will probably cause a number of deaths. For example, in the name of protecting the Earth's ozone layer, the EPA plans to ban most of the so-called metered-dose inhalers used by asthma patients because they contain chlorofluorocarbons, or CFCs. "It's another cynical exploitation of kids for the sake of environmental correctness," says George Washington University neuroscientist Robert Goldberg, who points out that the inhalers account for less than 1.5 percent of the atmospheric chlorine believed to deplete the ozone layer.[19]

The American Medical Association wrote to the Food and Drug Administration, which joined with the EPA in proposing the ban on inhalers, that inhalers "can relieve symptoms, prevent emergency-room visits, and, in many cases, they can be life saving."[20] Among other opponents of the proposal are most medical organizations, members of the Congressional Black Caucus who represent thousands of inner-city asthma sufferers, and members of Congress from both parties, including Representative Patrick Kennedy (D-R.I.), a chronic asthma sufferer — but not the APHA.

Manufacturers of non-CFC-using inhalers, as would be expected, supported the proposal, as did the American Lung Association, which has a long history of endorsing questionable products in return for financial grants from the corporations manufacturing the products.[21] But the ALA, like the APHA, also seems to be more concerned with environmental ideology than with the health of asthmatic children.

## A Scorecard of Political Correctness

The February 1997 issue of *The Nation's Health* included the association's "Annual Vote Tally" regarding "how members of Congress voted on issues affecting public health."[22] The resulting ranking of U.S. senators according to how their voting record matched the preferences of the public health establishment is illuminating. The senators were ranked according to their votes for funding for "international family planning," spending on environmental regulation, abortion training, medical savings accounts, price controls on health insurance, denying welfare benefits to *illegal* aliens, the balanced budget amendment, welfare spending in general, and partial-birth abortion.

Apparently, one must be far to the political left to promote "public health" as a U.S. senator, for the highest scores of 100 were given to Senators Barbara Boxer (D-Calif.), Diane Feinstein (D-Calif.), self-described socialist Paul Wellstone (D-Minn.), Frank Lautenberg (D-N.J.), and John Glenn (D-Ohio). Only Democrats received the highest scores by APHA, while only Republicans received the lowest. Senators ranked as "zeros" by APHA included Senators Murkowski (R-Alas.), Brown (R-Co.), Ashcroft (R-Mo.), Gregg (R-N.H.), Faircloth (R-N.C.), Inhofe(R-Okla.), Nichols (R-Okla.), Thurmond (R-S.C.), Gramm (R-Tex.), Hutchinson (R-Tex.), and Thomas (R-Wyo.).[23] Since these senators were all scored as "zeros" by the public health establishment, one can reasonably assume that, at best, their legislative efforts do absolutely nothing to promote the health of the American public and, at worst — the impression one gets from APHA literature — they most likely harmed it.

This political bias on the part of APHA has upset many of its members — public health professionals who do not share the ideological position that bigger government is the best route to improved public health. Such dissatisfaction is noted in periodic letters to the editor in *The Nation's Health*, but to no avail. For example, in an April 1996, letter Dr. Katherine Marconi of Middletown, Maryland asked, "Is there room left in APHA for health workers who are conservative or ... centrist?[24] APHA members come from the whole spectrum of political perspectives," Dr. Marconi felt compelled to remind the publishers of her profession's monthly trade magazine.[25] Despite the magazine's constant drumming of the theme of "diversity" in the work force and in society, it permits little, if any, diversity when it comes to the political or public policy agenda of the organization.

## "Presidential" Politics

Each issue of *The Nation's Health* includes an editorial from the association's president. The majority of these columns have little or nothing to do with pathology and public health, but are pleas for a greater politicization of society. One example is the frequent calls to extend government-enforced racial-hiring quotas in general and for the public health professions in particular. Former APHA president Caswell A. Evans, Jr. called for an "expansion of diversity in the public health work force" through quotas, arguing that "affirmative action ensures justice through equal treatment."[26] The APHA has joined with other political coalitions to oppose such policies as California's Proposition 209, passed in 1996 by a 56 percent majority in a state referendum, that forbids discrimination in state government hiring and university admissions on the basis of race, creed, color, religion, and national origin.

Common sense indicates that hiring public health professionals who are less qualified but of the politically correct race or gender would be harmful to health. There is mounting evidence that racial preferences have already severely diluted the quality of the medical profession. One study of twenty years of racial preferences at the University of California at Davis medical school found that "special admissions students performed strikingly less well than did the control group."[27] "Regular" admittees — that is, students of all races admitted on the basis of merit — were almost three times more likely to be admitted to the medical honors society than were affirmative-action admittees; with the latter group being eight times more likely to fail the National Board of Medical Examiners exams — a test that measures minimum competence in the core areas of medical science. No one who fails this exam may call himself a doctor.[28]

A 1994 *Journal of the American Medical Association* study also found that 51.1 percent of black medical students failed Part I of the exam (on core medical competence) compared to just 12.3 percent of white students, with racial preferences almost entirely to blame. When black medical students competed with white students with similar academic credentials they fared about the same.[29] Moreover, it is likely that medical students who only pass the exam on the third try after extensive tutoring are not likely to be able to keep up with the rapidly expanding base of medical knowledge in the future. Sending minimally qualified (or unqualified) minority doctors to practice medicine in minority neighborhoods — the objective of affirmative action proponents — is not doing those minority neighborhoods a favor. Nevertheless, to the APHA, politics apparently take precedence over public health.

The public health establishment's emphasis on politics is so powerful that it sometimes produces circular or contradictory the arguments. For example, in 1996 the EPA proposed stringent new clean air regulations to control airborne "particulate matter"— particles invisible to the naked eye. The EPA's proposal was based on some highly controversial research performed by EPA-funded researchers at the Harvard School of Public Health. The researchers refused to make their data public so that their results could be examined and replicated by other researchers, which raised questions about their political biases. Barry S. Levy, the APHA president, defended the EPA's position in refusing to make its data — paid for with tax dollars — public and subject to scientific scrutiny. In his July 1997 "president's column," Levy advised APHA members to support the EPA's position with the argument that "raw data often contain personal information on subjects and are routinely kept confidential."[30]

But at the same time the association issued an "Action Alert" to its members urging them to contact their senators and President Clinton to protest the "Family Privacy Protection Act" because the act "constructs barriers to the collection of integral public health data and poses a direct threat to the validity and reliability of federally funded public health research."[31] The act would require prior written parental consent for minors to participate in any federally funded survey or study. As such, the "Action Alert" warned that the act would undermine public health research by reducing participation rates in surveys, imposing supposedly onerous "burdens" on students who are asked to obtain written permission from their parents, and ultimately "obstruct the public policy process" that would lead to the implementation of the public health establishment's political agenda.

The public health establishment seems primarily interested in protecting the privacy of survey respondents when such protection suits its political purposes. It is not opposed to the invasion of personal privacy in principle, but as a matter of political expediency. This is not a trait of a scientific and scholarly organization, but of a special interest group.

At times the "president's column" borders on the absurd. In his March 1997 column Barry Levy posed a hypothetical situation — the year was 2072 and a public health professor was instructing his class on the history of the public health movement near the turn of the century. America in the late 1990s suffered from "inadequate health services for seniors," "more homicides than in other industrial nations," tens of thousands of people each year were dying of retrovirus infection, and death rates from many other diseases were increasing. Millions of children were suffering from "preventable diseases." The main cause of all these problems, the hypothetical professor argued, was capitalism: "Health care was increasingly provided by for-profit corporations."[32]

After being informed of these "facts," the students and their professor engaged in a "lively discussion," with the professor ultimately congratulating the young students for arriving at the "obvious" solution to all these problems caused by greedy profiteers: Public health professionals in the late twentieth century "could have set up a grass-roots advocacy training program and key alliances with other health organizations and with the women's, labor, environmental and other national movements."[33] Paraphrasing the title of Hillary Clinton's book, *It Takes a Village*, the professor concludes that "it really takes a society to practice public health."

In Mrs. Clinton's book, the word "village" is a euphemism for "government." Similarly, Dr. Levy's message is that it takes government control of the health care system to practice "public" health. Specifically, it takes the kind of government intervention created by a small number of special interest groups: the APHA, along with feminists ("women's groups"), labor unions ("labor"), environmental activists, and so on.

It is difficult to find any "president's column" during the past decade that did not contain political commentary. In his November 1996 column, for example, APHA president Richard Brown put forth a "public health agenda for children" that was filled with phrases like "encourage state initiatives," "develop a federal program," "support FDA regulations," "increase the excise tax on beer," "increase cigarette taxes," "ban alcoholic-beverage advertising," "raise the minimum wage," and "restore funding" to numerous federal programs while "rejecting efforts to mandate parental consent for a minor seeking family-planning advice."[34]

This litany of interventionism contains numerous proposals that have been proven policy failures for years, but are nevertheless accepted on faith by the public health establishment. Few things would be more harmful to the economic well being of the nation's youth than continuing to raise the minimum wage. It has been known for decades that the effect of the law is to price out of the market workers with the least skill and education — primarily teenagers and especially minority teenagers who disproportionately suffer from inadequate education.

Increased "sin taxes" on tobacco and alcohol will raise little revenue, will hardly deter smoking and drinking, and will give rise to black markets for those products, bringing children into contact with many of the same individuals who sell illicit drugs. The demand for cigarettes and alcohol is price inelastic — consumers do not reduce their consumption very much when prices increase. And if the taxes are sufficiently high, they will only create arbitrage opportunities for those who engage in the black market activity of purchasing untaxed cigarettes and alcohol — perhaps in Mexico or elsewhere — and selling the smuggled items more cheaply than the heavily taxed items.

The APHA cites Canada as an enlightened example of cigarette taxation after it raised taxes by $3.00 per pack in the early 1990s. But the artificially inflated price of cigarettes created such a profit potential for cigarette smugglers that smuggling quickly became rampant and organized crime came to dominate the smuggling trade. The Canadian government was forced to rescind the tax increase.

Banning advertising of alcohol and tobacco products is a recurring theme. And, several recent articles in *The Nation's Health* report that an increasing number of Americans, according to opinion polls, are in favor of gun control laws. That the public health establishment refers to opinion polls to make its case against the Second Amendment reveals its disdain of the U.S. Constitution. The whole purpose of the Bill of Rights, after all, is to place certain individual rights off-limits to majoritarian politics. It doesn't matter if a majority of voters wants to deprive some group in society of freedom of speech, religion, or self-defense. These are constitutionally protected rights, and it is government from which we are protected.

APHA presidents and others who write for the association's publications routinely list an impressive array of academic credentials next to their names: M.D., Ph.D., MPH, and so on. One would think that all this formal education would enable them to read and comprehend such things as the tables published in the *Statistical Abstract of the United States*, an extremely useful source of data on everything from government taxing and spending trends to international child mortality rates. But such is not the case. In their political appeals for higher taxes, more regulation, and bigger government, APHA presidents often get their facts wrong, even when the facts are readily available.

A case in point is former APHA president Eugene Feingold's 1994 plea for higher federal taxes in a column entitled "Paying the Price for Civilization." "During the Reagan Years," Feingold claims, "federal taxes were cut by 20 percent." But a quick look at the *Statistical Abstract* shows that during the "Reagan decade" of the 1980s federal tax revenues about doubled, as did the size of government. In 1980 federal government expenditures were $590.9 billion; by 1990 they had risen to $1.25 trillion, a 112 percent increase. Even by 1988, President Reagan's last year in office, revenues had increased by 80 percent, to $1.06 trillion.[35] Even after adjusting for inflation, federal *nondefense* spending increased by about one third during the "Reagan years."

## Political Action "Alerts"

Almost every issue of *The Nation's Health* contains at least one "Action Alert" urging APHA members to contact members of Congress and the president, write letters to the editor, join coalitions, and lobby for some kind of policy. "Action" is never urged in terms of educating the public about disease, spending more time on basic research, administering inoculations, and other necessary public health tasks. The "alerts" are exclusively political.

One 1993 "alert" wasn't a call for political action, but a celebratory announcement that President Clinton had abolished the Council on Competitiveness, the one office in the executive branch of government (within the Office of Management and Budget) that was charged with examining whether or not proposed regulations would in fact be likely to deliver public health benefits in return for the heavy costs — sometimes in the billions of dollars — that they would impose on American consumers and business owners. "APHA was one of the first organizations to oppose the [competitiveness] council," the announcement boasted.[36]

Each year there is an "action alert" to rally political support for increased governmental funding of abortions — both domestically and internationally. When members of Congress discovered that the Centers for Disease Control was funding lobbyist training seminars for proponents of gun control laws through its National Center for Injury

Prevention, APHA issued an "alert" asking readers to write members of Congress and remind them of how many gun-related injuries and deaths there are each year, as though those facts had anything to do with the use of tax dollars to illegally finance lobbying campaigns. Indeed, since the APHA is the recipient of federal funds, as are many of its institutional members, it was indirectly using tax dollars to lobby for the continued illegal use of tax dollars!

In fact, in 1995 the APHA lobbied against a bill by Representative Ernest Istook (R-Okla.) that would have been one of dozens of (rarely enforced) laws already on the books to prohibit the use of tax dollars for lobbying or other forms of partisan politics. "APHA has sent a letter to members of Congress in opposition to the amendment," an October 1995 article in *The Nation's Health* reported.[37]

The APHA has published manuals on political coalition-building and has organized various "coalition-building campaigns" in a number of states.[38]

A further indication of how completely wrapped up in politics the public health establishment has become is the APHA's Jay S. Drotman Award, given annually to "a health worker or student age 30 or younger who demonstrates potential in the health field by challenging traditional public health policy or practice in a creative and positive manner. Neither academic credentials or grades are a factor in the award."[39] This is quite a remarkable award, for it explicitly states that a student's grasp of knowledge of public health issues is not important — what counts is the students devotion to the political causes promoted by the association. One recent winner of the award was Joy Steinauer, a medical student at the University of California at San Francisco, who won the award for putting together a petition drive urging medical schools to do more in the area of "abortion training" and to "actively support abortion providers across the nation."

The APHA has also rallied its members to participate in the smoking prohibition movement, which epitomizes the shift in public health away from educating individual citizens on healthy lifestyles to relying on government coercion. An October 1995 "Action Alert" began in big black letters, "We need your help. Drop everything and write" your congressman.[40] The "alert" urged members to support the FDA's proposals to ban vending machine sales of cigarettes, limit advertising to a "tombstone format" (black and white text only), ban billboards in many areas, limit tobacco industry sponsorship of entertainment events, and require the industry to devote at least $150 million annually to be allocated by the U.S. Department of Health and Human Services on "public education" campaigns.

This money would constitute a gigantic windfall for the public health establishment, for who better to educate the public on health matters? This is also why the APHA has sent out numerous "action alerts" urging political support for a $2 per pack increase in the federal cigarette tax — it expects much of the revenue to be earmarked for programs administered by public health professionals.

It is doubtful that all those billions would be spent exclusively on programs to preach to teenagers the dangers of smoking. There have already been billions spent on such programs for decades and there is probably no one in the United States over the age of 10 who does not know that smoking poses serious health risks. Indeed, most Americans overestimate the risks associated with smoking, according to Harvard University economist W. Kip Viscusi, one of the nation's top experts in risk analysis.

Consequently, it is inevitable that such a large slush fund earmarked for the amorphous "public education" campaigning will be used to promote myriad other political causes promoted by the public health establishment, from gun control to extreme environmentalism to an enlarged welfare state.

No liberal cause goes unmentioned in the action alerts, from support for the 1992 "Earth Summit," to opposing the decentralization of regulatory powers to state and local governments, enhancing the budget and power of the EPA, expanding OSHA regulation, and on and on.

A 1997 action alert screamed that "public health safeguards are in danger!" The reason was a bill proposed by Senators Fred Thompson (R-Tenn.) and Carl Levin (D-Mich.) that would have required additional benefit/cost analysis and risk assessment in regulatory decision making. As mentioned in earlier chapters, with a fixed budget to be spent on public health improvements through regulation at any one point in time (assuming that regulation can actually improve public health), it is always wise to rank relative risks facing the public and to expend the most resources where the health risks are greatest. This is all that risk analysis tries to do, yet the approach is denounced by many public health professionals. In his July 1997 "president's column," for example, Barry Levy condemns risk analysis by declaring that deciding to spend tax dollars (or to force individuals to spend private dollars) to reduce one kind of health risk rather than another (i.e., more money for breast cancer exams, less for duplicative and ineffective "don't smoke" campaigns) is illegitimate because "this is not an either/or situation."[41]

But spending more dollars to reduce one kind of health risk necessarily means there are fewer dollars available to address other kinds of risks. That is why risk assessment is so important to regulatory decision making and why, thanks to the politicization of risk analysis by political pressure groups like the APHA, we have wasted billions of dollars over the past several decades on minuscule health risks while ignoring many larger ones.

## No Political Stone Left Unturned

The APHA seems to get involved in virtually every political issue facing Congress, and quite a few more that even Congress ignores. It has publicly called for an international ban on land mines, the cessation of nuclear testing, the creation of 1930s-era government-financed "jobs" programs, regulation of guns as a consumer product, targeting welfare more to the benefit of women (as though women live independently of men), prohibiting winemakers from advertising the well-established health benefits of moderate wine consumption, promoting unionism, banning certain types of alcohol advertising, limiting the ability of teenagers to work after school, publicly condemning the Republican party's "Contract with America," raising the minimum wage, and, "long troubled by the impact of a profit motive in health care," the association lobbies constantly for onerous taxes and regulations on private health care providers in a thinly veiled campaign to hamper their role in the market.[42]

Many of these issues are of questionable value to American public health. They are nevertheless promoted as "societal" cures. The next chapter discusses how the politicization of science in the public health field has created an aura of scientific respectability around many of these "cures" that is entirely undeserved.

# 8

# Political "Science"

*"The arts of power and its minions are the same in all countries
and in all ages. It marks its victim; denounces it; and excites the
public odium and the public hatred to conceal its own abuses and
encroachments."*
—Henry Clay, Speech, U.S. Senate, March 14, 1834

Public health research is almost exclusively funded by taxpayer
dollars, although a small percentage is also financed by private foun-
dations, such as the Robert Wood Johnson Foundation. Because of the
hostility toward capitalism harbored by many public health professionals, as discussed in earlier chapters, industry-funded research is
automatically discounted by many public health researchers as "biased"
and "suspect."

Oddly, these same researchers do not accept the notion that their
own research may at times be biased because of their reliance on government funding. This is odd because of the widely acknowledged fact
that political controls of one form or another are always attached to all
forms of government spending, including research spending.

This does not necessarily mean that all government-funded research
is corrupted by politics; much of it is of high quality. But it is inevitable that political pressures will systematically affect some government-funded public health research.

Public health research is particularly susceptible to politicization.
Many of the leaders of the public health movement consider themselves to be political activists, first and foremost, and they seek to use
their research funding to support their activism. There is nothing inherently "wrong" about using one's research to advance one's social or
political agenda; the point is that there are considerable pressures and
temptations to "cook" the data and to make unsubstantiated claims that
tend to cloak political agendas in the mantle of science. There is simply

too much money coming from government — billions of dollars per year — to public health research for it *not* to become significantly politicized.

## Political Incentives

In his book, *Science Funding: Politics and Porkbarrel*, Joseph P. Martino, a senior research scientist at the Research Institute of the University of Dayton in Dayton, Ohio, argues convincingly that special-interest politics poses a serious danger to the integrity of science in America.[1] Martino catalogues how political criteria are routinely used to establish research funding priorities and how members of Congress attempt to micromanage the funding of science, often freezing out innovative ideas in favor of "big" projects in which as much "pork" as possible can be ladled out to research institutions (primarily universities) in individual congressional districts.

For example, members of Congress routinely pressure administrative agencies (whose budgets they control) to fund "research centers" at many universities, even when there appears to be no good scientific reason for the grants and contracts. The universities quickly caught on to this practice, and now hire hordes of lobbyists to descend on Capitol Hill to retrieve their "share" of the science-funding porkbarrel: "In 1983 and 1984 together, Congress appropriated $100 million for laboratories and research projects solely on the basis of lobbying by the recipients. There were neither requests by the government agencies directed to spend the money nor congressional hearings on any of these appropriations."[2] The National Science Board warned that a "dangerous precedent" was being established by this politicization of science funding on the grounds that "funds were diverted from other scientific activities that had been selected on the basis of their merit" and "could well threaten the integrity of the U.S. scientific enterprise."[3]

The *content* of scientific research is also heavily influenced by politics as well. Since government does not have unlimited resources with which to fund scientific research, priorities must be established, and political considerations often override scientific merit. A clear example of this is the enormous success of AIDS researchers in procuring funding for "their" disease that is all out of proportion to the number of people who are affected by it compared to other diseases, such as cancer and heart disease.

The government's National Institutes of Health dispense funds for research on numerous diseases, each of which has its own nonprofit sector lobbying organization — the American Lung Association, American Cancer Society, and American Heart Association, for example. These organizations all lobby vigorously for what most Americans would agree are good causes. The point, however, is that such lobbying efforts will inevitably redirect science funding to those diseases which are associated with the most clever lobbyists, not necessarily the biggest public health threats.

The competition among researchers for government funding — and among government agencies that fund the research for congressional appropriations — has become so intense that questionable health "threats" are frequently "reported," all of which are supported by dubious "research." A particularly blatant example is the cancer scare of the 1970s that turned out to be nonexistent.

In her book, *The Apocalyptics*, Edith Efron recalled how, during the 1970s, *Time* magazine warned that cancer "would emerge from the industrial system"; Dan Rather of CBS News dramatically claimed that "we are suffering a cancer epidemic in slow motion"; and the *New York Times* wrote ominously of "a monstrous epidemic of occupational cancer."[4] These apocalyptic claims were all based on numerous studies, many of which were government funded, which claimed that hundreds of industrial products, from scotch whiskey to caffeine, diet sodas, and even children's pajamas, "caused" cancer.

One problem, however, is that there never was any "epidemic" of cancer that coincided with industrialization. In 1977 the World Health Organization reported that in most countries of the world (including the United States), "death rates were either stationary or declining"; in 1978, the National Center for Health Statistics reported that "death rates from all causes [of cancer] had *decreased* during the years 1940 to 1976" (emphasis added); in 1979 the American Cancer Society reported that the "overall incidence of cancer has decreased slightly in the past 25 years"; and in 1982 a National Research Council committee said that "the overall age-adjusted cancer rates have remained fairly stable over the past 30 to 40 years."[5]

Efron also discovered that the hundreds of false claims about alleged man-made carcinogens tended to come from people who had an ideological bias against capitalism — many of whom were environmental "activists" and held positions in government agencies. Most scientists knew that the claims were false when they were first made. Before her book was published Efron sent the manuscript to twenty of the top cancer researchers in the world. *Every one of them* praised the book. The claims of a cancer epidemic allegedly caused by industry was a case of an anti-capitalist ideological crusade funded with tax dollars and carried out by various segments of the public health profession.

It is an inherent feature of the incentives that exist within governmental organizations that agencies which fund public health research will frequently exaggerate the health risks of various phenomena. It has long been widely known that every government bureaucrat is inherently an empire builder, and fabricating public health "scares" such as the phony cancer scare of the 1970s — has become an ideal technique for garnering political support for bureaucratic empire building — and increased budgets to alleviate the "crises."

An agency that can succeed in creating the perception of an imminent public health threat stands to have its budget greatly enhanced and its powers expanded; money and power are the coins of the realm in politics. This is not to suggest that there are no genuine public health threats; there clearly are. The point is that minor or false threats are all too often presented to the public as dire emergencies that require the showering of tax dollars on the government agencies that fund public health research.

Politicians can also advance their careers by politicizing public health research. One tried and true practice is to support research that greatly exaggerates a threat; this enables the politician, the bureaucrat, and the "scientists" to take credit for championing governmental programs to reduce the nonexistent threat. For example, during the 1980s numerous politicians demanded that all asbestos be removed from every public school building in America, based on a deeply flawed study that has since been repudiated. There never was an asbestos "threat" in reality, but quite a few political careers were made by convincing voters that there was one and that only their elected officials could save them and their children from it. To this day the asbestos removal business is a multi-billion-dollar-a-year enterprise.

The asbestos scare was created by an *anonymous* report made public by the National Cancer Institute in 1978 that listed asbestos as a possible carcinogen.[6] The Manville Corporation, the nation's largest manufacturer of asbestos, went bankrupt, and the EPA banned all uses of asbestos by 1997.

But when legitimate scientists (as opposed to the EPA's anonymous ones) began researching asbestos, they found that the 1978 report "was so grossly in error that no argument based on it, even loosely, should be taken seriously."[7] That was the conclusion of renowned cancer researchers Richard Doll and Richard Peto. "There is no evidence that environmental exposure to asbestos is a public health hazard," concluded Yale Medical School's Dr. Richard Gee.[8]

A similarly bogus episode involved the public health scare over the chemical Alar, which is sprayed on apples to preserve their freshness. It was claimed that Alar was linked by "researchers" to cancer, which caused widespread panic among parents, whose children were fed apples and apple juice in school. Tons of apples were destroyed, thousands of gallons of apple juice were dumped down the drain, and the apple industry reported losses in the hundreds of millions of dollars. Then it was revealed that the "study" was hopelessly flawed; Alar has not been linked in any way to cancer. As the Advisory Committee on Pesticides for the British government concluded, "Even for children consuming the maximum quantities of apples and apple juice, subjected to the maximum treatment with daminozide [Alar], there is no risk."[9]

In fact, the Alar scare impaired public health by discouraging people from eating fruit, something that dietary researchers say can help deter cancer and other diseases.

So-called secondhand smoke is another public health scare that has led to hundreds of smoking bans throughout the U.S. and has fueled litigation. But the science behind it (discussed in more detail below) is extraordinarily weak—so weak, in fact, that in the summer of 1998 a federal judge in North Carolina ruled that the U.S. Environmental Protection Agency's "studies" of secondhand smoke were contrived, fatally flawed, and an inappropriate basis for public policy.[10]

### Tricks of the Trade

The politicization of public health research has become so pervasive that Steven Milloy, the director of Science Policy Studies at the National Environmental Policy Institute, has written a tongue-in-cheek handbook for public health "hustlers" who want to pervert public health science in order to promote their own careers.[11] *Science without Sense: The Risky Business of Public Health Research* is humorous in tone, but its substance is not. Milloy is the author of several books on risk assessment and has lectured widely and testified before Congress on the subject. He was motivated to write the book by his observation that despite the fact that the average American lives well into his seventies, and that the average life span is rapidly approaching eighty, "there are more public health professionals finding more public health problems than ever before."[12] Thanks to the "political entrepreneurs" in the public health profession, says Milloy, "public health has struck it rich — to the tune of billions of dollars in annual revenues."[13]

Milloy claims that his book is "an unabashed guide to using risk assessment to climb the public health career ladder" by playing fast and loose with the scientific method. His cynical writing style is entertaining, but the book nevertheless exposes a number of disturbing truths about the politicized path that too much public health research has taken.

One of the most frequently used tricks used by public health researchers is to study a risk that is unprovable. For example, the federal government's Superfund program to clean up hazardous waste sites has the criterion of cleaning up sites where one's risk of getting cancer is 1 in 10,000 or more. But "this risk is so small that it could never be scientifically shown to exist. It would take a study with at least 500 million subjects . . . to prove [that] such a small risk exists . . . the typical study [however] contains just a few hundred subjects."[14]

The "advantage" of this approach is that one can never be proved wrong (or right). Among the "health risks" that have been hyped by public health researchers who have utilized this trick are dioxin, electromagnetic fields, hazardous waste sites, secondhand smoke, household radon, chlorinated drinking water, and pesticides, to mention just a few.

Other "advice" that Milloy offers to the ambitious, but unscrupulous, public health researcher is to study risks that are ubiquitous, like electromagnetic fields or radon or chlorinated drinking water. People cannot escape these things, and they are more likely to panic if they can be convinced that they are risky.

"Good" risks to study should also be intuitive to the public, such as smokestack emissions, even if the emissions do not really cause any health problems. They should also be involuntary, such as electric power lines, the location of which cannot be controlled by average citizens. And they should be ones that other people (i.e., businesses) are responsible for, not ones that we are all responsible for, such as the food we choose to eat.

Perhaps the predominant means of playing fast and loose with statistics is to claim that a statistical *association* connotes *causation*. This kind of "cooking" the data to get politically correct results is especially prevalent in studies of "relative risk." So-called case-control studies compare the prevalence of exposure to a particular risk, like a high-fat diet, among disease victims (e.g., heart-disease sufferers) to the prevalence of exposure to the risk among a control group. Thus,

$$\text{Relative Risk} = \frac{\text{Prevalence of exposure among disease victims.}}{\text{Prevalence of exposure among control group.}}$$

If one performs such an analysis for the above-mentioned example and obtained a relative risk of say, 6.0, the proper interpretation of that number is that the incidence of heart disease in the case group was six times higher than in the control group. It does *not* say that the study shows that the risk of heart disease is six times higher for those with a high-fat diet, however that might have been defined in the study. But that is exactly what many public health researchers do: They argue cause and effect when in reality there is no statistical (or other) evidence of cause and effect.

All sorts of bizarre "relationships" can be obtained by this misuse of risk analysis by public health researchers. For example, one study found a relative risk of 2.14 for drinkers of whole milk and lung cancer; another study found a relative risk of 12,500 for those who wear brassieres all day and breast cancer; and yet another found a relative risk of 1.5 for the consumers of tap water and miscarriages.[15]

This misuse of risk analysis has been very effective in creating a sense of hysteria among some segments of the public over such things as environmental tobacco smoke (relative risk of 1.19 for lung cancer), olive oil (relative risk of 1.25 for breast cancer), coffee (relative risk of 1.3 for "premature death"), mouthwash (relative risk of 1.5 for mouth cancer), yogurt (relative risk of 2.0 for ovarian cancer), and myriad other products.[16]

Milloy also points out the incredibly sloppy techniques of data collection in many public health studies. The biggest problem in many of the studies (some are discussed below) is that *actual* exposure to health risks is never even determined. Survey data are used whereby people are asked if they can recall their degree of exposure to a risk (e.g., tobacco smoke, smokestack pollution, etc.) ten, twenty, or more years ago. Sometimes studies are published in peer-reviewed public health journals that are based on risk exposure surveys of *the relatives* of the people exposed to the risks, such as the children of deceased women whose husbands smoked. Such survey studies purport to examine the effects of environmental tobacco smoke on now-deceased women by relying on the memories of the women's children regarding events that occurred decades ago, perhaps when the children were in elementary school. The EPA used thirty studies of environmental tobacco smoke to make its case for banning smoking in public areas despite the fact that *not one of the studies even attempted to measure actual exposure* to secondhand smoke.

There is a built-in bias in such surveys. Milloy recalls one study of lung cancer victims who were asked if they were exposed to unusual amounts of diesel exhaust. Many of the cancer patients were eager to blame their health problems on that particular cause, so their responses were not likely to be very accurate. Nevertheless, public health researchers have published studies of the alleged cancer threat from diesel exhaust.

So-called "disease clusters" are another source of bogus public health threats. The incidence of diseases such as cancer is not evenly distributed among the population. One in three Americans will develop cancer at some point in his or her life, although this rate is higher in some parts of the country and lower in others. But as the geographic area gets larger the differences in cancer rates between areas narrow or disappear. The existence of so-called cancer clusters is essentially meaningless.

But public health researchers have ignored this statistical truth in order to fabricate cancer scares over alleged cancer clusters associated with hazardous waste dumps, electrical wires, the incidence of breast feeding, the use of hair driers, black-and-white television sets, incense, exposure to spray paints during pregnancy, and even hot dog consumption.[17] These studies are notoriously sloppy, for they do not (nor could they) control for the various other possible causes of the incidence of disease, including perhaps the most important cause: heredity. They are public health fishing expeditions that needlessly frighten the public.

Finally, far too much public health research ignores the first principle of toxicology that "the dose makes the poison." For example, it is well known that people exposed to massive doses of radiation, such as the victims of Hiroshima and Nagasaki, suffered horrendous health effects. It does not follow, however, that minuscule doses of radiation, such as the kind we get from x-rays, exposure to the sun, or naturally occurring radon in the home, poses any health risk at all. Yet, public health researchers have asserted that minuscule exposure to such things as radon is the equivalent to massive exposure and have given this theory the name, "linear nonthreshhold model." But such models defy common sense. After all, vaccines for polio, measles, mumps, diphtheria, and other diseases *improve* health by exposing people to low levels of toxins.[18]

## Smoke and Mirrors

Dozens of federal and state government agencies allocate billions of dollars annually for research in the "war" against smoking.[19] Much of this research is published in the *American Journal of Public Health* and in other peer-reviewed public health journals. And much of it is biased, unscientific, and political in nature. No one argues that smoking is not dangerous — but informed public policy regarding the health hazards of smoking (or of anything else) depends on sound research.

One of the most blatant examples of sloppy science in the service of politics is the Environmental Protection Agency's research on secondhand smoke. As mentioned above, a federal judge in the summer of 1998 ruled that that research, on which numerous smoking bans and lawsuits have been based, was so deeply flawed that it was essentially useless and should be disregarded.

The EPA declared secondhand smoke a possible carcinogen in 1993 based on an extraordinary manipulation of the data involved in numerous studies of the phenomenon. The first thing that the EPA did was to apply the "linear nonthreshhold model" by asserting that since it is known that cigarette smoking is linked to cancer, environmental tobacco smoke must also be. This may sound plausible, but the cigarette smoke that a smoker inhales into his or her lungs is not even remotely similar (chemically) to the smoke inhaled by a nonsmoker. As Dr. Gary Huber of the University of Texas Medical Center explained in the July 1991 issue of *Consumers' Research*, "ETS [environmental tobacco smoke] is so highly diluted that it is not even appropriate to call it smoke."[20] That is, nonsmokers breathe in only minute quantities of residual chemicals from environmental tobacco smoke. And since so many of the chemical compounds in tobacco smoke are unstable, it is not safe to assume that a nonsmoker is even exposed to the same chemicals that a smoker is.

Furthermore, even if secondhand smoke was analogous to smoking, it is not clear that such small doses could have an effect on health. The dose makes the poison. Professor James Enstrom, an epidemiologist at UCLA, estimates that someone regularly exposed to ETS takes in the equivalent of three cigarettes per year, and no studies have ever been done on the effects of such low doses of tobacco smoke on cancer.[21]

The EPA's 1993 "finding" was based on thirty epidemiological studies that compared lung cancer rates among nonsmokers, mostly women, who lived with smokers to lung cancer rates among nonsmokers who lived with other nonsmokers. *None* of the thirty studies attempted to measure actual exposure to ETS; the data were based on surveys of the memories of the subjects or, in cases where the subjects had died, of their relatives. This is bound to hopelessly confound the data and the results. A nonsmoking woman who truthfully told the researchers that she was never exposed to ETS at home would be counted as such. But the researchers have no way of knowing whether she worked eight hours a day in a smoky restaurant or bar, whether her close friends smoked, or if she was exposed to ETS elsewhere.

Of the thirty studies, only six indicated a statistically significant *correlation* between exposure to ETS and the incidence of lung cancer. By convention, epidemiologists call a result significant if the probability that the event occurred merely by chance is 5 percent or less — a 5 percent "confidence level." But the EPA used an unconventional 10 percent confidence level in order to get the results it wanted from the studies, thereby doubling the likelihood that the statistical associations were caused by mere chance.

Even after the data were massaged in this way, only one U.S. study found a statistically significant relationship and even that study was insignificant at the 5 percent confidence level. Since the EPA clearly intended to prove a preconceived notion rather than test a scientific hypothesis, it then applied what Steven Milloy calls the "mixmaster technique"— meta-analysis or case/control studies to determine "relative risk." The EPA also excluded from its analysis other studies published in 1992 that found no statistical link between ETS and lung cancer.[22]

Once the case/control studies were completed a relative risk of 1.19 was calculated, which enabled the EPA to broadcast around the world that women who live with smokers allegedly have a 19 percent higher chance of contacting lung cancer than those who live with nonsmokers. But such comments are unjustified for the same reasons that so much other talk of "relative risk" by public health researchers is: The studies do not account for a host of confounding factors — other things that may be the causes of lung cancer to which the women had been exposed. There are at least twenty other variables (other than tobacco smoke) that have been identified as "important to the development of lung cancer," according to Dr. Huber, yet none of them was taken into account in any of the EPA studies.[23] "Statistical associations found between disease and passive smoking could be incidental or misleading," the Congressional Research Service concluded in a masterpiece of understatement.[24]

Even by the EPA's own standards for relative risk studies, the ETS studies did not qualify as an important health risk. The agency routinely states that any relative risk below 3.0 is more or less inconsequential. By contrast, the relative risk ratio for male smokers is 20.0.

Clearly, the dissembling that plagued the presentation of research on ETS by the EPA was motivated by the desire to promote what EPA bureaucrats and public health researchers believe is a worthy cause: achieving a "smoke-free society." They apparently believe that this is a worthy cause even if it comes at the cost of the corruption of science.

## Dust-in-Your-Eyes Science

Another example of the politicization of public health is a proposal by the EPA to enhance its own regulatory reach (and its budget) by giving itself new authority to regulate so-called particulate matter — microscopic particles in the air that are invisible. A crackdown on such matter, the EPA claims, can possibly save 15,000 lives per year (revised downward from its earlier assertion of 20,000).

EPA administrator Carol Browner repeatedly asserted during 1997 and 1998 that voluminous research supported her proposal to strengthen EPA regulations on particulates, including even more stringent regulation of automobiles, industry, and, lawn mowers. But the research that allegedly links "particulate matter" with lung ailments is very unorthodox and highly questionable. Almost all of it — at least all of it that is cited by the EPA — has been done by the same three researchers, all of whom are funded by the EPA or have worked there (C. Arden Pope, an economist at Brigham Young University, and Joel Schwartz and Douglas Dockery of Harvard University). Dozens of contradictory studies are simply ignored by the EPA, and the three researchers funded by EPA refuse to make their data public even though the data gathering was financed by EPA grants, that is, by the taxpayers.[25] These three, according to science writer Michael Fumento, who has written a book about their research, "get lots of grant money, publish lots of papers, and almost invariably find positive correlations between particulates and sickness. But time and again, when other researchers attempt painstakingly to verify their results, they find they cannot do so."[26]

For example, Pope made a big splash in media and public health circles with a 1989 article in the *American Journal of Public Health* which purported to find a correlation between hospital admissions in Utah County, Utah, and particulate matter. This work, says Fumento, is "the bedrock of the EPA-environmentalist position" on particulate matter.[27] But there are major problems with it. Dr. Joseph Lyons of the University of Utah has explained that every other year there is a breakout of viral bronchiolitis in the Utah Valley, which raises hospital occupancy rates dramatically. This is what Pope's study picked up, not the effects of particulate matter, Dr. Lyons wrote in the 1996 *Journal of Pediatrics*.[28] Researchers at the National Institute of Statistical Sciences in Research Triangle Park, North Carolina, confirmed Dr. Lyons's research, but this work is largely ignored by the public health movement and by the EPA.[29]

In addition to simply ignoring the powerful evidence that the Pope study is fatally flawed, the public health movement politicizes the use of relative risk analysis when it comes to particulate matter. After a major study suggested that women who had had abortions suffered a 50 percent increase in breast cancer incidence, the federal government's National Cancer Institute declared that such a risk was "small" while the American Cancer Society dismissed it as only "a modest elevation" of risk.[30] But when particulate matter is said to create a relative risk of lung ailments of 5 percent, a crisis approaching a national emergency is declared and the EPA asks to be given the power to impose tens of billions of dollars annually in regulatory costs on the economy to ostensibly reduce this risk.

Armed with generous EPA grants, Pope, Schwartz, and Dockery have published studies of various cities that always seem to have the "correct" results — a link between particulate matter and lung ailments is found. And in every one of these cities, other researchers have failed to replicate their results or have discovered serious problems with their methodology and interpretations. Perhaps the most serious problem with the studies is that these three researchers rarely take into account the possibility of other causes of rising hospital admissions. According to Dr. Suresh Moolgavkar of the Hutchinson Cancer Research Center in Seattle, Washington, a fatal flaw in the EPA-funded studies is that "only one pollutant is observed at a time," whereas pollution is a complex process that involves more than just so-called particulates. Often times, says Dr. Moolgavkar, the researchers have access to data on other pollutants but fail to use it.[31]

In a widely cited study of six American cities, these three authors declared that in Steubenville, Ohio, which had the most air pollution of the six cities, the mortality rate was 26 percent higher than in Portage, Wisconsin, the cleanest city in their study. This result was broadcast far and wide by the EPA and by the news media. But a part of the study that was not broadcast was the part that explained how, when the researchers included only nonsmokers in their data sample, their results disappeared, as they did when they included persons with occupational exposures to gases, fumes, and dust.

Thus, it is likely that what they were measuring were the health effects of smoking or occupational dust, not of particulate matter. The EPA's public relations juggernaut nevertheless promoted these questionable results.[32]

These episodes prove an important point about the politicization of public health: Whenever government involves itself on one side of a policy debate, it has the capability of drowning out all other voices. This is especially true when the principal opponents of a policy are business people who can be easily demonized as concerned about profits and not health — the "greed" syndrome. This perhaps explains why EPA-funded researchers can get away with refusing to make their data public so that their research results can be checked by independent (and not-so-independent) researchers. When pressed on why he steadfastly refused to release his data, Professor Schwartz revealed a deep anti-business animus by explaining to the *Wall Street Journal* that he didn't want to turn over his data to "industry thugs."[33]

## Public Health Disease Mongering

In her book, *Disease Mongering: How Doctors, Drug Companies, and Insurers Are Making You Feel Sick*, Lynn Payer, a medical journalist who writes for the *New York Times*, argues convincingly that the medical profession, the nonprofit health charities, insurance companies, and the pharmaceutical industry profit by making us believe that we are sicker than we really are.[34] According to Payer the "cholesterol scam" costs us millions while actually making many people *less* healthy; much surgery — as much as 78 percent of cardiac surgery according to one study — is supposedly unnecessary; doctors routinely order unnecessary medical testing — and charge handsomely for it; the dangers of breast cancer, although very real, have been greatly overblown; and pharmaceutical advertising, and the industry's influence over the medical profession, have allegedly caused us to become a dangerously overmedicated society.

The public health movement — especially the executives of the APHA— would undoubtedly cheer Payer's book, for it is a condemnation of profit seeking as much as anything. It is the quest for profit that Payer believes is the root cause of "disease mongering." Take the profit out of health care, the public health movement argues, and such abuses will not occur.

Such an argument is questionable, however, for private-sector medical professionals cannot hold a candle to the public health movement in terms of fabricating phony health scares and exaggerating public health risks. It is a myth that government-run health care will magically transform the people who manage such a system into self-sacrificing angels who have no concern for money and profit. But the pursuit of money — in the form of tax dollars for bureaucratic budgets and re-search grants — is the driving force behind the corruption of public health science. Payer's book is not quite the condemnation of for-profit medicine that it might, at first glance, appear to be. A large part of the reason why so many unnecessary tests and procedures are performed is government intervention in the form of Medicare and Medicaid and the tax exemption of employer-provided, but not individually purchased, health insurance. Third-party payments through Medicare and Medic-aid have isolated millions of Americans from the process of shopping for health care services and products. Why shop when it's "free"? Con-sequently, health care providers are artificially given much more lati-tude in determining the kind of health care products that will be of-fered and what their prices are than would be the case in a genuine free market.

The tax exemption of employer-provided health insurance is the rea-son why most Americans are out of the loop in terms of the act of purchasing health care — it is purchased for them by their employers. A genuine free market in health care would eliminate the elements of socialism — Medicare and Medicaid — that exist in the current sys-tem along with making individually purchased health insurance tax exempt.

That said, it is worth noting that the whole purpose of the politicization of public health science is to expand the size and scope of the government agencies that sponsor this shoddy "research," to advance the careers of politicians and bureaucrats in the public health field, and to provide millions of dollars in research grants to govern-ment-funded researchers. It is *all* about money and power.

Lynn Payer's well-taken arguments about the private (but heavily regulated) health care market in no way imply that such problems do not exist in the public health field, for they certainly do, and are arguably even worse. As Steve Milloy pointed out, diminishing returns affect public health as much as any endeavor. Huge advances in public health were made in the late nineteenth and early twentieth centuries, as discussed in chapter 2. Advances continue, but they no longer have the dramatic effects on mortality and overall health that they once did. But at the same time the public health profession — heavily subsidized through government grants to schools of public health — continues to graduate more and more professionals.

The problem is that there is not quite the need for all these public health professionals that there was a century ago. Payer blames "too many doctors" for the "disease mongering" that occurs in the private practice of medicine. The same can be said for the public health profession: Too many government-funded public health professionals has created a situation where there exists a sort of disease-of-the-month club based on questionable research and multi-million dollar publicity campaigns.

It has long been a tenet of the scientific method that scientific discovery is an *ongoing process*. Research results provided by a single study are never "conclusive" if, indeed, any collection of results are. There is always a chance that someone will discover a superior theory or provide conflicting evidence. After all, in the field of statistics or epidemiology we can only speak in terms of probabilities, not of scientific certainty.

This tenet, however, is routinely ignored in much public health research. It has become common for a government agency to fund a researcher or a research team and include in the grant the funds required to conduct a public relations campaign to trumpet the "results" far and wide. The PR campaign is often begun after the publication of a single article in the *American Journal of Public Health*, the *New England Journal of Medicine*, or elsewhere. A scientifically uninformed media dutifully report the results — or at least the spin on the results that is offered by the researchers or the funding agency. This maximizes the chances that the single study — even if it is "peer reviewed" (by other government-funded researchers, typically!) — will become the basis for public policy changes desired by the funding agency.

A good example of this phenomenon is a very influential study by Stanton Glantz, a professor at the School of Medicine at the University of California at San Francisco whose doctoral degree is in applied mechanics but who publishes mostly in the area of political science. The paper, "The Effect of Ordinances Requiring Smoke-Free Restaurants on Restaurant Sales" (with Lisa Smith), published in the July 1994 *American Journal of Public Health*, purported to show something that is completely counterintuitive — that restaurants would not lose money if they barred a sizeable segment of their clientele — smokers — from their restaurants.

The paper was (and still is) accompanied by a massive, government-funded publicity campaign and consequently became the basis of dozens of local government ordinances which banned smoking in restaurants. A sure indication that Glantz and Smith were wrong, however, is the fact that in California, where smoking bans are statewide, there has been massive civil disobedience by restaurant and bar owners who have observed first hand the *decline* in their profits when the smoking ban was enforced. There have been numerous media reports of bartenders working beside signs announcing the statewide smoking ban while handing bar patrons ash trays.

The Glantz/Smith study was funded by the federal government, although it should be judged on its scientific merit, not necessarily the self-interest of the funding bureaucracy or the grant recipients. The same is true of a critique of the study by economist Michael K. Evans, the founder of Chase Econometric Associates and a Professor of Managerial Economics and Decision Sciences at Northwestern University. In a study that was funded by the National Smokers Alliance Professor Evans carefully examined the Glantz/Smith study and found that their handling of the data was quite sloppy.

For example, in their study Glantz and Smith claimed that fifteen "test cities" had 100 percent smoke-free restaurant ordinances. Checking on this claim, Evans found that in reality only one of the cities had such an ordinance.[35] In the other fourteen cities anti-smoking ordinances permitted smoking in free-standing bars and the bar areas of restaurants and cocktail lounges as well as in private function rooms, unenclosed patios, and separately ventilated rooms. Also, Glantz and Smith chose numerous "control cities" which, they asserted, had no smoking bans. Evans found that this was not true. Some restrictions did exist in some of their "control" cities, which means they were *not* comparing restaurant sales in smoking versus smoke-free restaurants, as they claimed. Evans believes that more than half (eight) of the control cities were misclassified.

Evans replicated the statistical technique used by Glantz and Smith after correcting for these flaws in the data gathering and found that in the twelve cities for which adequate data were available, nine of them

showed a *negative* impact on sales (of about 5 percent) from the impo-
sition of smoking restrictions. He concluded that "in virtually every
city where Glantz and Smith alleged [that] a smoking ban was imposed, there was a significant decline in sales of eating and drinking
establishments."[36]

Next to anti-smoking legislation, gun control laws are probably the
favorite policy of public health professionals because of their almost
"religious" belief that the government could somehow get rid of the
more than 200 million firearms that exist in the United States today,
thereby virtually eliminating gun-related violence. Such an event is, of
course, pure fantasy that any thinking individual would question. Yet,
it is an article of faith of the public health establishment which publishes myriad peer-reviewed articles "proving" that gun control laws
are necessary.

Typical of such studies is an article in the June 1997 issue of the
*American Journal of Public Health* entitled "The Association between
the Purchase of a Handgun and Homicide or Suicide" by five medical
doctors.[37] All such studies receive considerable notoriety in the media,
which tends to favor such laws.

The study is a typical relative risk study and a virtual caricature of
the problems of such studies cited by Stephen Milloy. A case-control
study of members of a health-maintenance organization was performed
where some of the case subjects were suicide or homicide victims. The
authors claim that there is a relative risk of suicide of 1.9 for persons
"with a history of family handgun purchase" and 2.2 for homicide.
They conclude that "legal purchase of a handgun appears to be associated with a long-lasting increased risk of violent death."[38]

The word "appears" is obviously a fudge factor. Since they are doctors and not social scientists, one cannot be too hard on these authors
for ignoring *all* other possible determinants of suicide and homicide
and controlling for *no other* potential causes in their study. But then
again, three of the authors possess masters degrees in public health,
and social science methods are taught in schools of public health.

They also ignore the benefits of gun ownership, in terms of offering
self-protection and personal safety, which have been shown in other
studies to save far more lives than are lost due to gun violence committed by criminals. Nor do they say anything about the criminal backgrounds or mental health of the people in their sample who committed
crimes with a handgun. Including violent criminals or mentally ill persons in their sample of handgun owners would surely bias their results,

but no such controls are even mentioned. Ignoring such controls is about as valid as taking a survey of "typical" or "average" sex practices by interviewing federal prisoners who had been convicted of sex crimes, as was apparently the case in the famous "Kinsey Report" on American sexual behavior that was published in the 1950s — not a proud moment for public health research.

Nor was any attempt made to control for varying degrees of criminal penalties for crime that might act as a deterrent. This is not unexpected, for most advocates of gun-control laws seem to believe that punishment is a weak or nonexistent deterrent to criminals. Yet, they *simultaneously* cling to the notion that criminals will obey the law if handguns are made illegal. The legal deterrent will work in the case of handguns, even if it doesn't work in other situations. The "logic" defies comprehension.

Sometimes the attempt by public health researchers to make political correctness sound "scientific" turns out to be quite humorous. Such was the case in a very impressively presented study in the March 1997 issue of the *American Journal of Public Health* entitled "Condom Breakage and Slippage during Heterosexual Intercourse: A French National Survey," which had no fewer than thirty-one co-authors![39] Loaded with statistical tables and scientific jargon, the article discusses a French survey of condom usage by 4,820 men and women. "Univariate analysis," when "entered simultaneously in a logistic regression model" resulted in the stunning scientific result that "high frequency of intercourse was associated with [condom] breakage but not with slippage."[40] Thank goodness for that valuable scientific knowledge.

Despite the old folk wisdom that "everyone lies about sex," these thirty-one government-funded research scientists assure us that "self-reports of recent condom failure are believed to be reliable, as are reports of recent sexual events in general."[41] The policy conclusion is that since condom breakage is rare among people with "more than 3 years of condom use experience" the study "provides supportive evidence for the appropriateness of condom promotion policies for youth."[42] Thus, in the name of improving the health of the nation's youth, these authors are saying not only that promiscuous sex is not something to be discouraged (they are French, after all), but it is actually safer the more one participates in it as long as one becomes proficient at avoiding "condom breakage." The authors offer no tips on how one might avoid such unfortunate and potentially lethal incidents.

Closer to home, a September 1997 study published in the *American*

*Journal of Public Health,* authored by six Ph.D. researchers and funded by the Robert Wood Johnson Foundation, the Aaron Diamond Foundation, the New York Community Trust, and the William T. Grant Foundation, reported on a survey of over 7,000 New York City school children who were asked detailed questions about their sex lives[43] ("Have you ever had any form of sex?" "Oral intercourse (mouth)?"; and "anal intercourse (anus)?"

After performing some very fancy statistical footwork the authors conclude exactly what their funding sources — promoters of condom distribution in schools — want them to conclude: that distributing "free" condoms in schools does not encourage students to become sexually active. Counterintuitive as this conclusion is, the biggest problem with it is that it is completely unwarranted in light of the fact that it is based on a single study which utilizes notoriously unreliable survey data taken from teenagers who were asked very intimate and embarrassing questions in school. Normally, scientific researchers would take a step back and note these drawbacks before making policy proposals. One rarely observes such modesty in the public health literature, especially in the pages of the *American Journal of Public Health.*

## Political Commentary Masquerading as Science

The *American Journal of Public Health* cleverly combines political commentary with research papers, thereby creating the impression that the commentary is based on science (since it appears in a peer-reviewed scientific journal). There is a place for political commentary — television and radio talk shows, newspaper op-ed pages, political magazines, and so on. We should all encourage and welcome such commentary as a healthy ingredient of a free society. But such commentary in an ostensibly scientific publication seems more likely to miseducate and confuse the public than enlighten it.

In the October 1997 issue of the *Journal,* for example, a lawyer named Scott Burris claims to "model" what he calls the "prevailing political attack on government."[44] His main point is that a market economy is "itself a major source of ill health." He offers no evidence of this, only polemical assertions. Indeed, he could not, for as mentioned in earlier chapters the evidence is overwhelming that wealthier economies tend to be healthier, and free-market capitalism is undeniably the surest route to economic growth and health improvement. Mr. Burris is contemptuous of individual responsibility and freedom of

choice, however, and makes a case that government should control virtually all lifestyle choices in the name of "public health." In "Women's Agenda
for Equality," published in the March 1996 issue, former APHA president
Helen Rodriguez-Trias reports on the 1995 World Conference on Women
that took place in Beijing, China.[45] The paper reported on all the various
liberal policy prescriptions that came out of the conference on women in
Beijing, where, incidentally, women are forced to undergo abortions in the
ninth month of pregnancy if it is discovered that they are about to give birth
to a female child that is in excess of the Chinese government's one-child-
per-family policy. Male children are not aborted as often.

In Beijing, the capital of a country that is governed by a communist
dictatorship, the conference issued a proclamation urging all governments to respect human rights. In addition to that, we are told that the
conferees championed abortion and opposed war, the beating and mur-
dering of women (but not men), and infanticide. These, of course, are
things that all civilized people would endorse regardless of whether or
not thousands of women from around the world went on government-
funded boondoggles to China to state them. The odd thing is why they
are discussed in a scientific journal that is ostensibly aimed at expanding our scientific knowledge. Their only purpose seems to be to assure
the readers of the *Journal* of the moral "superiority" of the activists within
the public health movement, such as Mrs. Rodriguez-Trias.

The *Journal* also includes periodic articles that are little more than
political cheerleading. One such article is a February 1994 article entitled "The Need to Mobilize Support for the Wellstone-McDermott-
Conyers Single-Payer Proposal," which was a proposal for government-
controlled medical care that was far more extreme than even the Clinton
administration's convoluted scheme. Then there's the December 1994
article by APHA president Eugene Feingold on "The Defeat of Health
Care Reform: Misplaced Mistrust in Government" and the July 1997
article cataloguing "The Activities and Influence of Public Health Advocates" (i.e., lobbyists) with regard to national health care reform.
The article concluded, not unexpectedly, that "the biggest barrier to
promoting pubic health in the 103rd Congress" was the failure to pass
a bill to nationalize the health care system in America.[46]

## Conclusions

We do not argue that *all* public health research is politicized. Our
point is that ever since the public health movement was transformed

into a political movement on behalf of various liberal causes during the 1960s, there have been many political activists in the public health movement who have become much more adept at public relations than at health science and that they routinely make claims regarding their published research that are simply not tenable. Consequently, we have been subjected to an endless stream of questionable public health "scares," from Alar to dioxin, asbestos, secondhand smoke, and electromagnetic fields, to name but a few examples. The unfortunate consequence is that because of the actions of a segment of the public health movement, the public is now warranted in being extremely skeptical of *all* claims made by public health researchers.

# 9

# Pawns and Mascots

*"The gods visit the sins of the fathers upon the children."*
*—Euripides, Phrixus (Fragment 970)*

As discussed in earlier chapters, nationalized health care is the primary long-run objective of the public health movement in America. No matter what the public health problem is, some form of government intervention always seems to be the "solution." One tactic or strategy that is employed to promote this government-control agenda is to pick certain segments of the population and treat them as political pawns or, as economist Thomas Sowell calls them, mascots, who are portrayed as pathetic or needy people whose problems ostensibly "justify" nationalized health care. Children are currently being used in this way in the context of proposals for nationalized maternity care which amount to nothing but the nationalization of children.

## Nationalized Child Care

The public health movement's case for nationalized child care (euphemistically called "universal maternity care") is laid out in a 1992 book published by the American Public Health Association entitled *A Pound of Prevention: The Case for Universal Maternity Care in the U.S.*[1] The first paragraph of the book bemoans the fact that too much responsibility for child rearing in the U.S. is assumed by parents and too little power is given to the government in the form of providing "social supports and health services."[2]

No one denies that there are problems related to childhood diseases, malnutrition, child abuse, and other maladies. But to the public health movement the only possible approach to solving these problems is nationalized child care: "If we are to improve the quality of life for young families . . . an important first step . . . is universal access to maternity

117

and infant health services."[3] And government-run child care would truly be universal, meaning "universal eligibility for all services without means testing and without out-of-pocket payments."[4] Ideally, according to the public health movement, everyone in the country — including illegal immigrants — should be eligible for an "extensive array of social supports and income benefits associated with pregnancy and childbearing: paid absences from employment for clinic visits, paid maternity leaves, birthing bonuses, family allowances, transportation privileges, housing benefits, assured day care, job protection, and home visiting by workers who counsel, instruct, arrange follow-up medical appointments, and even help with the shopping and housework."[5]

Think about this. Every family in the country, regardless of income, would be eligible for taxpayer-funded social workers who will even do their shopping and housework for them. Three observations are important here. First, such a scheme would require employing an army of additional social workers, which would balloon the ranks (and the dues revenues) of the American Public Health Association and necessitate massive tax increases.

Second, such an open-ended entitlement would impose tax costs that would likely make Medicaid and Medicare costs look trivial by comparison. "Most analysts"— none of whom is identified — supposedly "advocate . . . increasing taxes" for nationalized child care.[6] The government child care bureaucrats would constitute a potent political lobbying force for the expansion of the program and would constantly lobby for higher taxes in the name of "saving the children." Opponents of the tax increases would be demonized as heartless and selfish and unconcerned about the plight of "our" children. These gargantuan tax burdens, in turn, would make it all but impossible for average families to independently take care of their own children.

Third, such a system would create a massive moral-hazard problem. With highly paid government bureaucrats taking responsibility for all aspects of child health, many parents would be seduced into doing less and less *for themselves and their children*. Why bother if the state will do it all for you? Some parents will resist this temptation, but many will not. This will lead to more and more charges of parental "child neglect," which the newly created child-care bureaucracy will then seize on as a reason for an even greater expansion of its powers and budget — perhaps even for taking more children away from their "neglectful" parents.

The epidemic of fatherless children would be made even worse as irresponsible men who are inclined to abandon the women they have impregnated or their newborn children will be even more likely to do so if they can be assured that the women and children will be cared for generously. Their sense of guilt or shame will be greatly diminished, to the detriment of their children and the children's mothers.

The APHA book on "universal maternity care" invokes some very questionable statistics to help make its case. Contrary to the experiences of almost everyone, the book claims that government-run public health clinics provide better prenatal care than do private physicians. It cites a North Carolina survey of women on Medicaid where there were 11 deaths per 1,000 live births, compared to Medicaid women served "largely" by private physicians where there were 15 deaths per 1,000 live births.[7]

The problem is that visits to a clinic are assumed to be *the sole cause* of infant mortality rates and that the four percentage point difference in the rates is caused by that one factor alone. But before one can jump to that conclusion one would have to investigate the overall health of the women in the two categories. A woman's own health is the most important determinant of infant mortality; a few visits to a government-run clinic may have only a marginal effect, if any effect at all. As is the case in so much of the "political" science invoked by the public health movement, these dubious statistics are discussed as though they are indisputable scientific truths.

As with so many other policy proposals that emanate from the public health movement, the proposal for nationalized child care is informed by a crude, simplistic, and vaguely Marxist view of the economic world. Wealth and income are not viewed as things that are earned through work, saving, investment, and entrepreneurship, but are just "out there" as a part of "society's resources." Consequently, the problem is that "important structural changes have occurred in the means by which society funnels its assets."[8] "Society's" assets — not the privately owned assets of individual members of society — are somehow "funneled" to children. "The great tragedy of children in America," the APHA's book continues, "is that their claim to justice is inherently tied to that of their parents. Social concern for children is framed by the fact that their access to societal resources depends on the legitimacy of their parents' claim."[9] Again, income does not belong to those who earned it, but to "society." The denial of the legitimacy of private property is the essence of socialism.

The political cat is let out of the bag in one of the essays in the APHA book in which Paul H. Wise says that "to argue for enhanced prenatal care services without a purposeful strategy to advance the cause of enhanced access to health services for all women regardless of child-bearing status is to cling to an isolated elevation of the children's claim and a rejection of a shared agenda."[10] Translating from the public health bureaucrat's idiom into plain English, this means that once national-ized child care is achieved, the next step in the political strategy is to point out how unfair it is that childless women are without a compa-rable array of "social services." Nationalized health care should cer-tainly extend to them, too, and to fathers, men without children, and all other permutations of the population until "universal health care" is achieved. The very last paragraph of the APHA book explicitly states this agenda: "the United States will adopt new social policies affecting women and children gradually. In the meantime, [universal maternity care] is a substantial first step toward a comprehensive approach to our children's future."[11]

In the concluding chapter of *A Pound of Prevention,* Jonathan B. Kotch and Rosemary Barber-Madden describe an "ideal" system of nationalized health care. A new federal "Bureau of Maternal and Child Health" would be created, putting the federal government "officially" in charge of monitoring the health of everyone's children. Maternity care "trust funds" would be set up in each state, financed by a new Medicaid-style federal tax; new taxes on insurance companies, em-ployers, and uninsured individuals; and the Social Security Trust Fund would also be raided.[12]

Any private-sector health care providers would be strictly regulated by the new federal bureau and by new state government bureaucracies staffed by legions of new public health bureaucrats and regulators. All of this bureaucracy is somehow supposed to lead to greater cost efficiency.

No one would be permitted to legally spend any of their own funds on extra care, for to "permit the purchase of premium supplements" would be to invite "insidious discrimination."[13] These authors disdain any and all kinds of inequality. Even if parents would like to spend more of their own incomes on caring for their children, they would be prevented from doing so under this "ideal" plan, because the plan's authors want the government to assure that "all infants . . . start out with equal opportunity" in health care.[14]

Ideally, one would think that it would be a *good* thing to encourage parents to work, earn, and save in order to provide better lives — including better health care — for their children. But this proposal would drasti-cally curtail such incentives — and diminish the health of many children. Spending one's own money on health care for one's own children would mean "inequality" and should therefore be prohibited.

## Do Children Really Need More Government?

The cause of nationalized maternity care is driven more (perhaps exclusively) by ideology than by facts. The federal government recently evaluated a pilot program for "child development" known as the "Comprehensive Child Development Program."

Created in 1988, the program was modeled after a Chicago program called "The Beethoven Project." The idea was "to provide intensive social services to poor mothers for the first five years of their children's lives. They would get everything from parenting classes to job training to drug counseling. . . . Young mothers received home visits every two weeks from 'case managers,' who taught parenting skills, advised on personal problems and identified useful government services."[15] About 4,000 families were enrolled.

The program sounds almost exactly like the one put forth in *A Pound of Prevention*. The government forecast that with its help mothers would become better parents and their children would thrive. If the program worked on a small scale, then a case would be made to go national — to implement nationalized child care for the entire country. But it didn't work. The government contracted with the consulting firm Abt Associates to evaluate the program, and the firm concluded that the program "did not produce any important positive effects on participating families."[16]

Comparing participating families to a control group, Abt Associates found that after five years 40 percent of the mothers in the program had found jobs, but 41 percent of the control group did too; weekly wages were almost identical in the two groups; exactly 68 percent of each group was on food stamps; children in each group visited doctors at the same rate; and the children scored almost identically (81.1 and 81.0) on the Peabody Picture Vocabulary Test.[17]

In other words, the program was another huge waste of money; the families would have done just as well (if not better) without all the "social services." But perhaps Abt Associates is using the wrong criteria here. In terms of providing lucrative job opportunities for public health social workers, and fattening the membership roles and dues revenues of public health trade associations like the APHA, the program was a "success" and will therefore be vigorously defended by the real beneficiaries of the program.

*Newsweek* and *Washington Post* columnist Robert J. Samuelson offered some wise advice on such programs when he wrote that one of the lessons that ought to be learned from this experience is that "the 'investments' that truly count for children come from parents: love and security, discipline and instruction, a sense of worth. But large federal programs . . . can't undo parental failure. Nor can they offset the ill effects of family breakdown."[18]

Worse yet, such programs create dangerous moral-hazard problems: "If society can 'invest' its way out of social problems, then individuals are relieved of responsibility. Marriage loses its social value. Young men can father and abandon children. Mothers and fathers can easily leave troubled marriages."[19] Samuelson notes that there were once powerful taboos against such behaviors, but they have been largely broken down by the interventions of the welfare state.

### Is There Really a Child Care "Crisis" in America?

In 1998 Hillary Rodham Clinton declared that America was in the grip of a "silent crisis" of child care (could it be "silent" because it is in fact nonexistent?). A White House Conference on Child Care was convened on October 23, 1998 which was attended by hundreds of public health experts, politicians, bureaucrats, union leaders, and academics.

The one thing all the participants seemed to have in common was that they would all personally benefit from a new federalized child care program. The politicians could claim credit for "solving" another "crisis"; public health bureaucrats would have billions in additional funds to spend; unions could sign up thousands of additional dues-paying members ("We need government and business to play a bigger role [in child care]," said AFL-CIO president John Sweeney); and academic researchers would reap a harvest of research grants.

According to reporter Pia Nordlinger, who covered the conference, it was essentially a forum for market bashing. Then U.S. Treasury Secretary Robert Rubin declared that "the market is dysfunctional" when it comes to child care.[20] "When it comes to child care, Adam Smith's invisible hand is all thumbs," another speaker announced to "hoots of delight and clapping."[21]

President Clinton proposed some $20 billion in federal subsidies for government-supervised child care programs, but his legislation was not enacted in 1998. Perhaps Hillary Clinton was right when she alluded to a "silent" child care crisis. A January 1997 survey by NBC

News and the *Wall Street Journal* asked Americans about the two or three most important issues facing the nation that they would like to see the government in Washington do something about. Only 1 percent said "child care."[22] This, of course, does not mean that the proposal is dead; there are too many vested interests devoted to carrying forward the agenda of nationalized child care who stand to benefit from large increases in federal expenditures.

There is also an ideological angle: Some advocates of nationalized day care admit that their main objective is economic equality for women in the workplace, not children's health. If only mothers were unburdened by their babies they would be more "equal" to men in terms of earning capacity in the marketplace. As one of the pillars of modern feminism, this view implicitly assumes that a mother's job of caring for her children is not very important and requires little real skill. That is why just about anyone (i.e., "professional" child care bureaucrats) is said to be capable of doing it. Consequently, millions of American women now drop off their infant children at institutionalized day care centers where their babies languish all day long with as many as several dozen (or more) other children, none of whom receives much genuine motherly attention. It has now been documented that day care has had many serious, detrimental effects on children. A nationalized program of "universal" government-run day care would only amplify these pathologies.

Centuries of experience, common sense, and an expanding volume of social science research has determined that virtually *all* forms of institutionalized child care, no matter how high the quality, are inferior to a mother's care. Moreover, institutionalized child care may cement in place certain deleterious qualities in virtually all children that may haunt them later in life. Government-run "universal maternal care," in other words, may very well be hazardous to children's health, but this possibility is rarely mentioned by the advocates of nationalized child care.

Researcher and writer Maggie Gallagher surveyed some of the medical and social science research on the effects of institutionalized child care and found the following results:[23]

- Children in full-time day care are less likely to be firmly attached to their parents and are less obedient to adults and more aggressive toward their peers than children raised primarily by their own parents and families;
- Group day care exposes babies to numerous diseases, especially respiratory infections that may affect them for life;

- Chronic ear infections are much more likely for children in group day care; these infections have been shown to have such long-term effects as permanent hearing loss, lowered IQ, poor school performance, and learning disabilities;
- One British study found that children placed in day care suffered from retarded language skill development; and
- A study of some two thousand couples over a 15-year period found that sons of women who worked more than 45 hours per week attained, on average, a full year less of education than sons of women who worked less (or not at all) and earned nearly $9,000 a year less.

Writing in the *Wall Street Journal*, social scientist Andrew Peyton Thomas reported the results of a similar literature review:[24]

- Children "raised" in institutionalized day care are more likely to be violent and anti-social;
- Day care increases the likelihood that a child will be verbally and physically abusive of adults; and
- A study of children raised in Israeli communes (Kibbutzim) were at significantly greater risk of developing schizophrenia and other serious mental disorders.

Some of the research on the health risks involved in group day care are shocking. Epidemics of diarrhea and related diseases routinely sweep through day care centers, where infants under one year of age have eight times as many colds and other infections as do children raised at home.[25] Dr. Stanley Schuman wrote in the *Journal of the American Medical Association* that day care centers are responsible for recent

> outbreaks of . . . diarrhea, dysentery, giardiasis, and epidemic jaundice — reminiscent of the pre-sanitation days of the seventeenth century. Other serious day care hazards include cytomegalovirus, shigellosis, hepatitis, HiB, and ear infections.[26]

The May/June 1998 issue of the *American Enterprise* included a long series of articles by various authors who have studied extensively or who have had much experience with professional day care (some as providers), and provided many words of warning about *all* day care, regardless of quality. Story after story was told of how, no matter how well credentialed, well meaning, and professional day care providers were, there are always serious problems with leaving infant children under the care of an institution. It is physically impossible for even the best day care providers to give small children the kind of personalized care that a mother can. This is not true of all children who enter day care, but it is a general tendency.

The advocates of nationalized "maternity care" admit that all these problems exist with day care, but then use those problems to make their case for a single, government-controlled, monopoly system of "quality" day care. That was the principal message of the 1998 White House Conference on Child Care, for example.

But such a proposal turns facts, history, and common sense on its head. Government bureaucracies are known for *anything* but quality and efficiency, for one thing. And "uniformity" (through regulatory regimentation) is just a synonym for "monopoly." In no other industries would any rational person insist that monopoly — and government-run monopoly at that — would lead to desirable results for the consumer. Yet, that is exactly what nationalized maternity care would be: a government-run monopoly.

The "monopoly" need not be a system of government-owned maternity care centers; the same thing can be accomplished by federal regulation that coerces all maternity care providers to behave as federal regulators want them to behave or risk fines or loss of license. But the very idea that establishing "national standards" through regulatory regimentation will improve rather than diminish the quality of day care is misguided. There is no universal definition of "quality" day care, nor could there be. Parents have diverse preferences and private sector day care providers have different ideas about how to best satisfy those preferences in the marketplace.

The reason that there currently exists a wide array of day care services is precisely because the marketplace is a success in catering to the divergent preferences of parents — some prefer professional day care and the instruction it offers, whereas others who are more concerned with personalized attention rely more on family members. Many parents want religious or cultural instruction; others do not. In any case, religious instruction would be effectively precluded in schools funded by government. Uniform standards mandated by the state could not possibly accommodate all these preferences. Such a system must necessarily substitute the preferences of government bureaucrats for the preferences of parents.

The market for day care services, like all markets, is an ongoing, dynamic process of constant and continual discovery. In the quest to please their customers (and to enrich themselves), successful day care providers are always on the lookout for ways to improve their services. Competition in the marketplace spawns innovation, but such innovation is stifled if there are universal regulatory standards, for fear that an innovation may run afoul of regulations.

It is inevitable that a government-controlled day care industry will be guided more by politics than by concern for children's welfare. For example, in 1998 President Clinton defined his own criteria for "quality" child care in terms of the degree of governmental accreditation, wages of child care workers, and levels of government funding, not the health and well-being of the children.[27]

Nor should it be expected that government-imposed standards would even necessarily improve quality at all. After all, licensing and regulation are already pervasive in the industry, and there are serious problems in many licensed day care centers. Furthermore, establishing a system of universal regulatory standards will essentially place a ceiling on quality, as day care providers are given strong incentives to meet the standards, but no more. And there is much evidence that politicians and bureaucrats will avoid closing down failing or fraudulent day care centers once they are a part of a federalized system because of the politically embarrassing ramifications. A *Washington Post* article documented how many of Washington, D.C.'s government-subsidized day care centers (subsidized by the federal Department of Housing and Urban Development) continued to receive government funding despite failing to meet minimal health and safety standards. Unlike private, unsubsidized providers, many government-subsidized centers stay in business no matter what.[28] Thus, government regulation can (and often does) give consumers a false sense of "quality."

Regulation and licensing also make day care more expensive, as does virtually all regulation. Consequently, it imposes financial hardships on some families while pricing other (lower income) families out of the day care market altogether.

The advocates of nationalized maternity care often claim that in Europe, where many countries do have nationalized day care, the quality of care is vastly superior to that in the U.S. In reality, the quality of nationalized day care is Europe is often mediocre, at best. The European country that spends the most on government-run day care is France. But even there the average day care center has one teacher or supervisor for every twenty-two children, rendering the centers mere custodians or warehouses.[29]

Belgium's day care system is almost identical system to that in France. In Belgium the average day care "instructor" has a high school education; many of them are people on welfare who, in return for their welfare check, are assigned by the government to work at a government-run child care center. On a typical day about one third of them do not show up for work. This is the "ideal" system the American advocates of nationalized maternity care point to as exemplary.

## An Experiment in Nationalized Maternity Care

In the fall of 1998 California voters narrowly passed by referendum the "California Children and Families First Initiative" that would attempt to establish a state government-run system of maternity care funded by a new tobacco tax. The initiative passed by a mere 13,000 votes out of a total of 8 million votes cast (0.2 percent). In addition to a new fifty cent per pack tax there is a 35 percent tax on the wholesale value of dealer inventories, which will force some merchants to pay tens of thousands of dollars in lump-sum taxes.[30] There is also a "surtax" of 2.5 cents for every cigarette distributed, payable by retailers.

The initiative was spearheaded by the actor and comedian Rob Reiner, best known as the character "Meathead" in the television series, "All in the Family," who had established a "California Children and Families First Foundation." The law was apparently drafted by Reiner and his lawyers, who purported to speak on behalf of all the people of California. The proposed law declared that "the people find and declare" that "there is a compelling need in California to create and implement a comprehensive, collaborative, and integrated system of information and services to promote, support, and optimize early childhood development from the prenatal stage to five years of age."[31]

In essence, the new law seeks to impose the state in family child-rearing affairs beginning before birth until age five, at which time the child enters the government school system.

As with virtually every government program, the advocates of this one claim that the expenditure of billions of dollars will save the taxpayers money in the long run by making children far more likely to succeed in school, a dubious proposition at best. Given the failures of the public schools — which are at a crisis stage in California — it is strange to entertain the notion that what is needed is to place children *more* rather than less in the hands of state and local government bureaucrats. Yet, that is the assumption behind the new law — that more bureaucratic control (and, consequently, less parental control) of children is needed.

The new program will hire thousands of new government bureaucrats to "educate" the public about "nurturing" under the assumption that all families — not just low-income families — are in need of educating on the topic of nurturing their own children. And while they are at it, the newly hired bureaucrats will also "educate the public . . . on the dangers caused by smoking," even though virtually everyone already knows that smoking is unhealthy and there are already dozens of federal and state government programs that spend billions of dollars annually on anti-smoking education. Californians will be creating tens of thousands of jobs for public health bureaucrats, but their success in improving the health of children is dubious.

The tobacco tax revenues that will be used to fund the program will not be placed in the general fund but in a separate "trust fund," placing them off limits from democratic control by elected state representatives. The program will also seek to monopolize the day care industry by imposing "appropriate standards" for all providers of maternity care. The act seeks to create "an integrated, comprehensive and collaborative system" and to "eliminate duplicate administrative systems."[32]

This means that the program will eliminate all *competition*, which is euphemistically referred to as "duplicate administrative systems" by the law. A massive new administrative bureaucracy will be created to accomplish the monopolization of child care services in California. A state California Children and Families First Commission comprised of seven political appointees would be created, which would fund and create county-wide commissions of similar nature. The county commissions is ostensibly where 80 percent of the funds would be spent according to the new law. Funds are to be distributed to the county commissions on the basis of the percentage of births recorded in the county in proportion to the total number of births in the state.

All employees of the commissions "shall be exempt from civil service," which will allow them to become involved in partisan politics (i.e., lobbying) while on the job, something which is forbidden for regular state and local government employees. Thus, a formidable lobbying force of state taxpayer-funded bureaucrats will be created, virtually guaranteeing that this new bureaucracy (and its budget) will grow far beyond what its advocates are today claiming.

The state commission will establish "guidelines" for all child-care providers to follow. The guidelines will be adopted after only a single public hearing. Once the guidelines are put into place there will be periodic evaluations, but since the evaluations will be conducted by the commission itself there is little chance that they will be objective or that any shortcomings of the program will be well publicized.

The new law itself imposes thirty-six regulatory "requirements" on county governments that are recipients of funds from the new state child care commission, and more regulations are sure to follow. As mentioned above, such requirements tend to increase the cost of day care, which will balloon the commission's budget well beyond its proponents' cost estimates. The program may well create a regulatory nightmare for day care providers, and it can only be amended by a two-thirds vote of both houses of the California legislature.

### What Kind of "Childhood Education?"

The advocates of nationalized maternity care — especially in California — are eager to take children at birth and have them "socialized" by "experts" in public schooling, public health, and other fields of social work. By definition, this kind of education would be different from the kind of education that children would receive from their own parents. The key question becomes, therefore, what kind of childhood education? Some likely answers can be obtained by examining what goes on today in primary education itself, for many of the same "experts" who now ply their trades in the public schools will presumably be involved in any new educational programs for preschoolers under a system of nationalized child care, such as the one being established in California.

Economist Thomas Sowell has researched what he has found to be pervasive "classroom brainwashing":

> A variety of courses and programs, under an even wider variety of names, have been set up in schools across the country to change the values, behavior, and beliefs of American youngsters from what they have been taught by their families, their churches, or the social groups in which they have grown up. . . . Schools [have] set sail on an uncharted sea of social experimentation in the re-shaping of young peoples' emotions and attitudes.[33]

For example, sex education classes are rarely about sex education per se, but about *re-shaping of attitudes* about sexual behavior in a politically correct way — in a way that is often very different from the attitudes taught to children by their parents, relatives, and churches. Sowell documents how in school program after program the objective is not primarily to provide students with information or to teach them to think independently and analytically, but to have them adopt the "proper" emotions.

Sowell's survey of psychological "conditioning" programs that exist in thousands of American schools is shocking, in that many of the programs seem to "use classic brainwashing techniques developed in totalitarian countries."[34] This is a strong statement, but Sowell backs it up with voluminous facts.

The first technique of classroom brainwashing, according to Sowell, is stress and desensitization. For example, public school children are routinely brought to morgues to view corpses; students in "death education" classes are asked to write their own obituaries, suicide notes, and to discuss deaths which have occurred in their families; and children are asked to decide which members of their families should be sacrificed in life-and-death situations, such as trying to survive in a lifeboat that cannot hold everyone.

In some sex education classes eleven-year-old boys are shown models of female genitalia, ostensibly to educate them on how tampons fit.[35]

In North Carolina, one child fainted when shown a childbirth movie that parents were told was a movie on "vitamins." Many other schoolchildren are shown explicit, pornographic movies after which they are quizzed about their own sexual "attitudes."[36] Other schools attempt to brainwash children into being in favor of unilateral disarmament in "nuclear education programs." Such programs rarely provide children with information on both sides of military/foreign policy issues; instead, their objective is to inculcate into children's minds the "proper" or politically correct attitudes.

Isolation and cross examination is the second brainwashing technique that Sowell found to be pervasive in American schools. Once children are placed under stress and "desensitized" to certain issues, they are then isolated from others who may share their values (i.e., the ones taught them by their parents). Schoolchildren are not physically isolated; they are just embarrassed and humiliated in front of their classmates for holding "improper" attitudes. In one school, "a junior high school girl was required to defend her religion and values under extreme ridicule from the group leader and from her peers."[37] In some cases, teachers ask a class how many agree with a recalcitrant student, using a menacing tone of voice to indicate to the class that they are not to agree with the student but with the teacher.

Stripping away defenses is a third technique. Sowell reviews school psychological programs whereby children are told to write diaries containing personal information about their family and then the information is shared with the class and the teacher. In one "values clarification" class students were expected to share their views on such questions as, "What disturbs you about your parents?" "Do you believe in God?" "How do you feel about homosexuality?" "Tell where you stand on the topic of masturbation." "Reveal who in your family brings you the greatest sadness, and why."[38]

The purpose of these exercises is apparently to obliterate the child's sense of his or her own unique personality so that their personalities can be more easily molded and manipulated. Portraying parents as pariahs seems to be a characteristic of most "values clarification" programs according to Sowell. Moral relativism is another primary objective. As one widely used sex education texts states: "Remember, there are no 'right' or 'wrong' answers—just *your* answers."[39]

Once children's natural psychological defenses are broken down and their individuality erased, they can then be brainwashed into believing the politically correct views — and only those views on everything from environmentalism to national defense policy, affirmative action, and welfare reform. Unable to think analytically about any of these issues, they are instead conditioned to emote over them, to develop a sense of moral superiority over those who disagree with their politically correct viewpoints, and to condemn as evil and cold hearted those who disagree with them.

There is a massive psychological conditioning industry that is at work in America's public schools with the objective of essentially eradicating many of the thought processes and attitudes children have been taught by their parents in their preschool years. Is it any wonder, then, that the advocates of nationalized maternity care are so anxious to get their hands on children the day they are born and begin to subject them to "proper" educational influence by "experts." If this can be accomplished then much of the brainwashing that currently takes place in grades K through 12 would be unnecessary.

### A Military "Victory?"

The advocates of nationalized maternity care point to the U.S. Army as a successful example of government-run maternity care which should be replicated in the civilian sector. At the 1998 White House Conference on Child Care a star panelist was Major General John G. Meyer, who had recently retired as the commanding general of the U.S. Army's

Community and Family Support Center. General Meyer boasted that 85 percent of the child care centers run by the Army were accredited by the National Association for the Education of Young Children, as opposed to the national average of just 5 percent.[40] "Commitment, Standards, and Funding" were the keys to the Army's success according to the general. In exchange for the loyalty of Army personnel to the state, the general explained, the Army takes care of their children.

The number of Army combat divisions was cut in half during the 1990s, but the service's expenditures on day care centers tripled, apparently signaling a new focus and function for the U.S. Army: social service provider.[41] There are over 800 day care centers operated by the U.S. Army, making it by far the largest supplier of child care services in the nation.

The Clinton administration *ordered* the Army to begin to proselytize the civilian world on behalf of government-run day care centers. The Army responded by producing books, videos, and seminars for corporations that may be lagging behind the Army's performance. "What we're hoping is that this model will be applicable in the civilian sector," Hillary Clinton told reporters at Quantico Marine Corps Base in early 1998.[42]

Such a transformation would have ominous implications for the family, for the explicit purpose of what is called the "Total Army Family" is to denigrate the traditional independent, self-reliant family and replace it with a collectivist version that is under pervasive state control. (Amazingly, the concept of a Total Army Family was first mentioned in George Orwell's book, *1984*).

Real families are said to be subservient to the Total Army Family, an essentially totalitarian notion reminiscent of Stalin's Russia or Mao's China in which the idea of autonomous families with rights of privacy was all but nonexistent. After all, the military is run on a command-and-control system whereby individual rights are intentionally ignored for the good of the whole. It is, in other words, a thoroughly collectivist institution.

Predictably, and despite the government propaganda about the "success" of the Total Army Family, there are severe problems with the families that have been socialized by the U.S. Army. For one thing there are abnormally high rates of family turmoil and divorce; young Army couples are 64 percent more likely to be divorced by age twenty-four than comparable civilian couples.[43]

Second, as is true in the civilian population, generous welfare benefits ladled out to Army families have subsidized family breakup; as many as 40 percent of military pregnancies occur among unmarried service people. Indeed, the military encourages illegitimacy by not requiring pregnant females to identify the fathers of their children.[44] And the sexual integration of the armed forces has created a virtual epidemic of illegitimate births, with Navy ships returning to port carrying expectant women in uniform.

Political scientist Allan Carlson explains why the Clinton administration and other supporters of nationalized maternity care have been such enthusiastic proponents of the Total Army Family concept and its application to civilians:

> Back in the 1930s, the Swedish theorist Alva Myrdal showed how radical feminism might be reconciled with a collectivist vision of "the family": women must be employed alongside men in the same jobs; marriage must be transformed from a social expectation into a mere "choice"; the costs of children should be subsidized by the state; and the very young should be raised collectively. Some commentators argue that American military family programs are mere parallels to civilian benefit plans. In fact, their whole logic rests on this model of Scandinavian socialism.[45]

The essence of the Total Army Family — and of nationalized maternity care in general — is an attempted governmental takeover of the family in an effort to use it to reengineer our society. It has little to do with improving the health of children.[46]

# 10

# From Pathology to Politics

*"The only real moral crime one man can commit against another is
the attempt to create, by his words or actions, an impression of the
contradictory, the impossible, the irrational, and thus shake the
concept of rationality in his victim."*
—*Ayn Rand,* Atlas Shrugged

*"Error of opinion may be tolerated where reason is left free to
combat it."*
—*Thomas Jefferson, First Inaugural Address, 1801*

In *The People's Health,* a "memoir" of the public health movement in
general and the Harvard School of Public Health in particular, science
writer Robin Marantz Henig celebrates the movement's transformation
from pathology to politics.[1] "The old public health days," Henig writes,
when finding an elusive pathogen was the primary concern, have been
replaced by the need to deal with issues that encompass nearly every
aspect of our lives, including race, ethics, economics, politics, sexual
and family behavior, genetic predisposition, social infrastructure, and
even . . . a population's belief in its own collective future."[2]

Henig, whose book is endorsed on the back cover by former U.S.
surgeons general C. Everett Koop and Julius B. Richmond, as well as
the New York City health commissioner and researchers at Harvard
and the Carter Center in Atlanta, sees the politicization of public health
as an unequivocal good. But a very different interpretation is given in
this book. Given our understanding of the political economy of bureaucracy, it is realistic to assume that the shift from pathology to politics has been detrimental to public health. The eradication of various
diseases (primarily due to the efforts of private medical researchers)
and the dramatic reduction in public health problems during the early
part of the twentieth century left people employed in the public health
movement wondering what was left for them to do. Like any bureau-

cracy, this one did not just "declare victory" and find another line of work. It decided that it was (and is) imperative to continue to "discover"— if not fabricate — new public health "threats."

In declaring such things as poverty, violence, maternity care, and "the social infrastructure" as "public health" problems, the public health movement has given itself a virtually unlimited domain of responsibility. It seems as though no matter what the problem, to the public health movement the "answer" is invariably to weaken the institutions of capitalism and to rely on government control and regulation. Indeed, reading the literature of the American Public Health Association, one gets the impression that its principal purpose is to serve as a political lobby for nationalized health and child care. To a very large extent the public health movement has increasingly become a collection of liberal ideologies cloaked in the language and garb of health science. This is not to suggest that there are not many public health professionals who are sincerely interested in solving public health problems, only that the leaders of the public health movement clearly view themselves as political activists first and health professionals second.

The public health establishment makes much of its past accomplishments, a half century or more ago, and justifiably so. And public health departments around the U.S. continue to provide many valuable services, from disease inoculation to water quality control. But most Americans are unaware of the dramatic and fundamental transformation of the public health profession that took place in the 1960s and which is recounted in chapters 3 and 4. The point of demarcation seems to have been in 1968, when the APHA embraced the federal government's Kerner Report on the "root causes" of poverty and announced that social policy, rather than public health, per se, would henceforth become its main focus.

There is nothing inherently undesirable with the APHA being involved in social policy with regard to health issues. Indeed, it is eminently desirable to have an association of health professionals help inform the public discussion and debate on such issues. The problem, as is discussed throughout this book, is that there is little, if any, debate *within* the APHA itself over competing approaches to social issues. The organization — and hence much of the direction of the profession — is now dominated by ideologues who are so far to the left that they even opposed the failed Clinton health plan, condemning it as "too market oriented."

The resources and prestige of the public health profession are routinely utilized to support social policies that have been long been discredited as failures. Thus, we have the APHA claiming that:

- Being on welfare is conducive to improving public health;
- Government income redistribution programs can improve public health;
- Individuals should *not* be held responsible for their own health (government should be);
- Welfare programs, not medical science, are the best way to eradicate disease;
- Inanimate objects, per se, such as bicycles, automobiles, and firearms, are hazardous to public health, not the way in which individuals use (or misuse) them;
- Government "jobs" programs can reduce unemployment, contrary to all historical evidence;
- Free market capitalism is generally hazardous to health, unlike socialism; and
- Nationalized health care is superior to a health care system dominated by private health care providers and insurers.

During the 1980s the APHA even actively supported the communist government of Nicaragua and continues to point to communist Cuba as a model of "enlightened" health care and education policy. Although it is absolutely correct that poverty leads to public health problems, the APHA's social and economic policy recommendations would only make poverty worse. For example, it favors "upward harmonization" of taxes and regulations as a prerequisite for free trade agreements. By reducing the domain of free trade such regulations would diminish economic growth and increase poverty. Indeed, as catalogued in earlier chapters, the APHA favors massive tax increases to fund nationalized health care and an expanded welfare state, as well as much more pervasive regulation of business in general, all of which would be harmful to economic growth.

The public health profession is also a key player in what might be labeled the "anti-industry industry."[3] For example, it participated in organizing the international boycott of the Nestlé Company in the 1970s and 1980s over the allegations that Nestlé's infant formula that was sold to third world mothers was unhealthy. The claim turned out to be false, but the episode was part of the public health establishment's ongoing efforts to discredit private sector entrepreneurs in order to advance the cause of nationalized health care.

For centuries, Americans have cherished their Second Amendment right to bear arms for personal protection, among other reasons. Thomas Jefferson himself championed the Second Amendment for this very reason and urged all citizens to become proficient in firearm use and safety. But in the name of "public health" the public health establishment has adopted a doctrinaire, pro-gun control position. There is room for disagreement among reasonable people over the efficacy of the proliferation of firearms, but no such disagreement seems to be tolerated by the public health establishment. This is why, when University of Chicago legal scholar John Lott published his book, *More Guns, Less Crime* in 1998, the initial response of the public health establishment was to denounce Professor Lott personally by accusing him of being a secret shill of gun manufacturers.[4] Even if this were true, however, Professor' Lott's research — which provides powerful evidence that gun ownership *reduces* violent crime — would still stand. The fact that the public health establishment chose to attack Professor Lott personally rather than criticize his research suggests that it is more interested in defending its political ideology than arriving at scientific conclusions about such important public health issues as gun violence.

Professor Lott's research concludes that states experiencing the largest reductions in violent crime are the ones with the fastest growth rates of gun ownership. Violent criminals are deterred when they know innocent citizens are capable of defending themselves. If Professor Lott is right about this and the public health establishment is wrong, then the establishment is, indeed, hazardous to the public's health.

We have also discussed the politicization of science in the public health movement. Although there is a great deal of sound science that continues to be produced by public health researchers, there are nevertheless numerous instances of the systematic "cooking" of data and misreporting of research results, as described in chapter 8. Sometimes the politicization of science takes on bizarre proportions, such as the "relative risk" study that reported that women who wear brassieres all day are 12,500 times more likely to contract breast cancer than those who go braless.

Many relative risk studies have been so frequently reported by the news media that they have become accepted truths among Americans, even though many of the studies do not even attempt to measure actual exposure to real risks. All too often the data in these studies are obtained through dubious questionnaires which ask people if they can recall their exposure to various risks decades ago.

There are serious children's health problems that are addressed by highly skilled public health professionals in America. But the public health *movement* seems to be primarily interested in its agenda for nationalized child care, not providing needed services to individual children. As discussed in chapter 9 the movement has been lobbying for years for "universal maternity care," a euphemism for nationalized child care run by the government. The movement's ultimate goal is apparently for the state to effectively nationalize the day care industry, either outright or through federal regulation and regimentation. A new "Federal Bureau of Maternal and Child Health" would be created and put in charge of monitoring the health and welfare of everyone's children. Such a proposal can only be described as Orwellian. In light of the kind of "brainwashing" that goes on in so many primary and secondary schools (to borrow a term from Thomas Sowell), one cringes to think of the mischief that could be done if the state were to "take control" of child care from birth to kindergarten.

In 1998 the Clinton Administration promoted the military's child care experiment as a "model" that should be replicated nationwide. The "Total Army Family" is what its proponents call it. To those who think that our use of the word "Orwellian" to describe these schemes for nationalized child care is too extreme, we again point out that the phrase "Total Army Family" was first used in Orwell's *1984*.

The public health movement decided long ago that individuals were not primarily responsible for their own health and well-being; the state was. That being the case, there are signs that the movement is seeking to have the government control more and more of our personal behavior. Recall that the rallying cries of the anti-smoking crusaders were that (1) some 400,000 Americans died prematurely each year due to smoking-related diseases, and (2) these deaths impose billions of dollars of health care costs on the rest of the public. These are the two principal rationales for the increased taxes and liability lawsuits imposed on the tobacco industry and for the $250 billion "settlement" reached in 1998 with the state attorneys general.

Even before the ink was dry on that "settlement," some of the most visible members of the anti-smoking movement began targeting the firearms and food and drink industries with nearly identical claims to the ones that were made against the tobacco industry. Former U.S. Surgeon General C. Everett Koop formed a political pressure group called "Shape Up America!" which began issuing press releases claiming that "in sheer numbers and its costs to society, obesity has reached crisis proportions in the U.S."[5] "From a public-health perspective," Koop continued, "this situation is nothing short of a crisis" as there are "300,000 premature deaths each year from obesity-related conditions."[6]

Moreover, the "costs attributable to obesity" included "$11.3 billion for Type II diabetes and $22.2 billion for coronary heart disease . . . $2.4 billion for gallbladder disease; $1.5 billion in treating hypertension; and $1.9 billion for breast and colon cancer therapy."[7]

Citing "researchers" who have been "able to calculate" these costs, Koop makes no mention of the fact that there are likely to be numerous causes of each of these diseases, not the least potent of which is heredity. Granted that obesity has been linked to all these diseases, it is simply not believable that it could be known with such certainty that every one of the premature deaths included in these estimates was caused, without any doubt, by one factor and one factor only: obesity.

The same argument was made about the 400,000 premature deaths figure repeated endlessly by the anti-smoking crusaders, but with no effect; when the public health movement is on a moralistic crusade it never lets facts and reason get in its way. Now, there is nothing undesirable about urging Americans to slim down, eat healthier, and get more exercise. But we hardly need C. Everett Koop to alert us to this; the culture is filled with dietary advice, exercise "gurus," and thousands of books and videos of every kind informing us about how to lose weight. That being overweight is unhealthy is just as well known as is the fact that smoking is hazardous to one's health.

What we are witnessing with these new appeals to "Shape Up America!" is a new tobacco-style political campaign to force us into politically correct consumption patterns by taxing "high-fat" food and drink, restricting advertising of "fatty foods," and "earmarking" some of the billions of tax dollars raised to ongoing crusades by the likes of C. Everett Koop to lecture and harangue Americans to "Shape Up!" in the name of "public" health.

Professor Kelly Brownell, director of the Yale Center for Eating and Weight Disorders, has advocated in the *New York Times* "taxing of low-nutrition foods" with a sliding scale of taxes whereby foods "would be judged on their nutritive value per calorie or gram of fat; the least healthy would be given the highest tax rate. Consumption of high-fat food would drop, and the revenue could be used for bike paths and running tracks."[8]

Brownell decries the fact that alcohol prohibition failed because of a "lack of political will," and wishes that it could be resurrected, along with the prohibition of tobacco. But until that occurs, "we realize they carry tremendous social burdens, so we tax them to increase the price and decrease the use. Why can't the same thing happen with food?"[9] Like so many other public health specialists, Brownell decries Americans' reliance on "individual responsibility," which he sees as a road-block to public acceptance of his schemes to manipulate society in his image through the tax system.

The denial of individual responsibility for one's own life and well-being has become the keystone of the public health movement. For if individuals are responsible for their own health, who needs the "public" health establishment's political agenda? The very word "public" in this regard is really a euphemism for "socialized." And once our health is socialized, than *all* behavior becomes the "legitimate" province of state control and regulation. But once it is agreed that the state has a "right" to control any and all behavior that might possibly have a negative effect on "public" health, then we are on the road to losing all of our privacy and our freedom. As Friedrich A. Hayek wrote in *The Constitution of Liberty*:

> Liberty not only means that the individual has both the opportunity and the burden of choice; it also means that he must bear the consequences of his actions. . . . Liberty and responsibility are inseparable.[10]

# Notes

## Chapter 1

1. Al Gore, *Earth in the Balance* (New York: Penguin, 1993).
2. See James T. Bennett and Thomas J. DiLorenzo, *The Food and Drink Police: America's Nannies, Busybodies, and Petty Tyrants* (New Brunswick, NJ: Transaction Publishers, 1998).

## Chapter 2

1. Jacob Sullum, *For Your Own Good: The Anti-Smoking Crusade and the Tyranny of Public Health* (New York: Free Press, 1998), pp. 62-63.
2. Mazyck Porcher Ravenel, ed., *A Half Century of Public Health* (New York: Arno Press, 1970), p. 4.
3. Marshall W. Raffel and Norma K. Raffel, *The U.S. Health System: Origins and Functions* (New York: Wiley, 1989), p. 263.
4. Mazyck P. Ravenel, "The American Public Health Association," in his edited volume, *A Half Century of Public Health*, p. 16.
5. Ibid., p. 21.
6. Ibid., p. 26.
7. Ibid., p. 103.
8. Ibid., p. 110.
9. Frederick L. Hoffman, "American Mortality Progress during the Last Half Century," in Ravenel, *A Half Century of Public Health*, p. 112.
10. Hugh S. Comming, "The United States Quarantine System during the Past Fifty Years," in Ravenel, *A Half Century of Public Health*, p. 120.
11. Ibid., p. 123.
12. Ibid., pp. 130-31.
13. Charles V. Chapin, "History of State and Municipal Control of Disease," in Ravenel, *A Half Century of Public Health*, p. 139.
14. Philip Van Ingen, "The History of Child Welfare Work in the United States," in Ravenel, *A Half Century of Public Health*, p. 303.
15. George Martin Kober, "History of Industrial Hygiene and Its Effects on Public Health," in Ravenel, *A Half Century of Public Health*, p. 409.
16. Raffel and Raffel, *The U.S. Health System*, p. 264.
17. Ibid., p. 31.
18. See James T. Bennett and Thomas J. DiLorenzo, *Unfair Competition: The Profits of Nonprofits* (Lanham, MD: Hamilton Press, 1989).
19. Clint Bolick, *Grassroots Tyranny: The Limits of Federalism* (Washington, DC: Cato Institute, 1993).
20. Raffel and Raffel, *The U.S. Health System*, p. 289.

143

21. Ibid., p. 296.
22. Ibid., p. 285.
23. Terry Anderson and P.J. Hill, *The Birth of a Transfer Society* (Stanford, CA: Hoover Institution, 1980), p. 44.
24. Raffel and Raffel, *The U.S. Health System*, p. 285.
25. Richard Epstein, *Takings: Private Property and the Power of Eminent Domain* (Cambridge, MA: Harvard University Press, 1985), p. 296.
26. American Public Health Association, *Public Policy Statements of the American Public Health Association, 1948-1994 Collection* (Washington, DC: APHA, February 1995).
27. Ibid., pp. 1-4.
28. Ibid., p. 3.
29. Ibid., p. 6.

# Chapter 3

1. American Public Health Association, *Public Policy Statements, 1948-1994 Collection.*
2. James Bovard, *The Farm Fiasco* (San Francisco, CA: Institute for Contemporary Studies, 1989).
3. APHA, *Public Policy Statements,* p. 33.
4. Ibid., p. 42.
5. Ibid., p. 61.
6. Ibid., p. 45.
7. Ibid., p. 81.
8. Friedrich Hayek, *The Road to Serfdom* (Chicago: University of Chicago Press, 1994), p. xxiii.
9. Sally Satel, "The Politicization of Public Health," *Wall Street Journal*, December 12, 1996.
10. Ibid.
11. Ibid.
12. APHA, *Public Policy Statements,* p. 83.
13. Ibid., p. 84.
14. Ibid.
15. Ibid., p. 110.
16. Ibid., p. 97.
17. Ibid., p. 46.
18. Charles Murray, *In Pursuit: Of Happiness and Good Government* (New York: Simon and Schuster, 1988), p. 131.
19. Nancy Krieger, Letter to the Editor, *Wall Street Journal*, January 3, 1997.
20. Richard E. Messick, ed., *World Survey of Economic Freedom, 1995-96* (New Brunswick, NJ: Transaction Publishers, 1996); James Gwartney, Robert Lawson, and Walter Block, *Economic Freedom of the World, 1975-1995* (Vancouver: Fraser Institute, 1996); and Kim R. Holmes, Bryan T. Johnson, and Melanie Kirkpatrick, eds., *1997 Index of Economic Freedom* (Washington, DC and New York: Heritage Foundation and Dow Jones Company, 1997).
21. Richard E. Messick, "Economic Freedom Around the World," *Wall Street Journal*, May 6, 1996.
22. Ibid.
23. Tom Carter, "Study Links Political, Economic Freedoms," *Washington Times*, May 11, 1996.

24. Messick, *World Survey of Economic Freedom*, p. 17.
25. Gwartney, Lawson, and Block, *Economic Freedom of the World*, p. xv.
26. Holmes, Johnson, and Kirkpatrick, *1997 Index of Economic Freedom*, p. xiv.
27. Ibid.
28. APHA, *Public Policy Statements*, p. 165.
29. Regina E. Herslinger and William S. Krasker, "Who Profits from Nonprofits?" *Harvard Business Review* 65 (January/February 1987), pp. 93-107.

# Chapter 4

1. American Public Health Association, *Public Policy Statements*, p. 312.
2. Ibid., p. 312.
3. Ibid., p. 313.
4. Ibid.
5. David Horowitz, *Radical Son: A Journey Through Our Times* (New York: Free Press, 1997), p. 350.
6. Ibid.
7. Ibid.
8. Ibid.
9. APHA, *Public Policy Statements*, p. 204.
10. Ibid., p. 176.
11. Ibid.
12. Ibid., p. 548.
13. Ibid., p. 177.
14. Ibid., p. 209.
15. Ibid.
16. Ibid.
17. John C. Goodman and Gerald L. Musgrave, *Patient Power: Solving America's Health Care Crisis* (Washington, DC: Cato Institute, 1992), p. 491.
18. Ibid., p. 492.
19. Ibid., p. 493.
20. U.S. General Accounting Office, *Canadian Health Insurance: Lessons for the U.S.* (Washington, DC: GAO, June 1991), p. 55.
21. Cited in Milton Friedman, *Input and Output in Medical Care* (Stanford, CA: Hoover Institution, 1992)
22. Ibid.
23. Ibid., p. 12.
24. Ibid.
25. Goodman and Musgrave, *Patient Power*, p. 503.
26. Ibid.
27. John C. Goodman, *National Health Care in Great Britain: Lessons for the USA.* (Dallas, TX: Fisher Institute, 1980).
28. Julian LeGrande, "The Distribution of Public Expenditure: The Case of Health Care," *Economica*, 45 (May 1978), pp. 125-42.
29. Goodman and Musgrave, *Patient Power*, p. 508.
30. Mary-Ann Rozbicki, *Rationing British Health Care: The Cost/Benefit Approach* (Washington, DC: U.S. Dept. of State, 1978), p. 17, cited in Goodman, *National Health Care in Great Britain*, p. 193.
31. Goodman, *National Health Care in Great Britain*, p. 196.
32. Ibid., p. 198.
33. Dennis Lees, "Economics and Non-Economics of Health Services," *Three Banks*

*Review* 110 (June 1976), p. 9, cited in Goodman, *National Health Care in Great Britain*, p. 199.

34. Lawrence Reed, "Free ... But the Patient Doesn't Get Well," in Jacob Hornberger and Richard Ebeling, eds., *The Dangers of Socialized Medicine* (Fairfax, VA: Future of Freedom Foundation, 1994), pp. 71-74.
35. "Mouse Terrorism," *Wall Street Journal*, June 9, 1997.
36. Wendy Gramm and Susan E Dudley, "The Human Costs of EPA Standards," *Wall Street Journal*, June 9, 1997.
37. Ibid.
38. Ibid.
39. APHA, *Public Policy Statements*, p. 272.
40. Ibid., p. 553.
41. Ibid.
42. Ibid.
43. Ibid., p. 531.
44. Ibid., p. 240.
45. Ibid., p. 400.
46. Ibid., p. 280.
47. Herman Nickel, "The Corporation Haters," *Fortune*, June 16, 1980, p. 130.
48. Ibid., p. 126.
49. Reported in Carol Adelman, "Infant Formula, Science, and Politics," *Policy Review* 23 (Winter 1983), p. 110.
50. Ibid.
51. Ibid.
52. Ibid., p. 114.

# Chapter 5

1. Lawrence Wallack and Lori Dorfman, "Media Advocacy: A Strategy for Advancing Policy and Promoting Health," *Health Education Quarterly*, 23 (August 1996), pp. 293-317.
2. Ibid., p. 295.
3. Ibid.
4. Ibid.
5. Ibid., pp. 293-94.
6. Ibid., p. 298.
7. U.S. Department Of Health and Human Services, Centers for Disease Control and Prevention, "National Violence Prevention Conference," (Washington, DC: HHS, 1995).
8. Injury Prevention Network Newsletter, Building One, Room 311, San Francisco General Hospital, San Francisco, CA 94110, funded by CDC grant #R49/CCR903697-06.
9. Ibid., Spring 1995.
10. Ibid.
11. Omnibus Consolidated Appropriations Bill HR 3610, Pub. L. No. 104-208. Centers for Disease Control and Prevention.
12. James T. Bennett and Thomas J. DiLorenzo, *Destroying Democracy: How Government Funds Partisan Politics* (Washington, DC: Cato Institute, 1985) and idem., *CancerScam: Diversion of Federal Cancer Funds to Politics* (New Brunswick, NJ: Transaction Publishers, 1998).
13. Arthur Kellermann, "Comment: Gunsmoke — Changing Public Attitudes Toward

Smoking and Firearms," *American Journal of Public Health* 87 (June 1997), pp. 910-13.

14. *San Francisco Examiner*, April 3, 1994.
15. Cited in Miguel A Faria, Jr., "The Perversion of Science and Medicine," *Medical Sentinel* 2 (Summer 1997), p. 84.
16. Cited in ibid., p. 83.
17. Cited in "MD's Ill Treatment," editorial, *Augusta Chronicle*, August 1, 1995.
18. *Journal of the Medical Association of Georgia*, March 1994.
19. *Augusta Chronicle*, August 1, 1995.
20. Don B. Kates and Henry E. Schaffer, "Public Health Pot Shots: How the CDC Succumbed to the Gun 'Epidemic,' *Reason* (April 1997), pp. 25-29.
21. Ibid., p. 26.
22. Ibid.
23. Ibid.
24. Ibid., p. 28.
25. Ibid., p. 29.
26. Ramsey Clark, *Crime in America: Observations on Its Nature, Causes, Prevention and Control* (New York: Simon and Schuster, 1970).
27. Daniel D. Polsby, "From the Hip," *National Review*, March 24, 1997, pp. 33-35.
28. Gary Kleck, "Crime Control Through the Private Use of Armed Force," *Social Problems* (February 1988), pp. 1-21.
29. Ibid.
30. See John R. Lott, Jr. "Childproof Gun Locks: Bound to Misfire," *Wall Street Journal*, July 16, 1997.
31. Wallack and Dorfman, "Media Advocacy," p. 293.
32. Sanford Levinson, "The Embarrassing Second Amendment," *Yale Law Journal*, 99 (1989), p. 637.
33. Alshil Amar, "The Bill of Rights As a Constitution," *Yale Law Journal* 100 (1991), p. 1131.
34. Joyce Malcolm, *To Keep and Bear Arms: The Origins of an Anglo-American Right* (Cambridge, MA: Harvard University Press, 1994), p. 209.

# Chapter 6

1. The Advocacy Institute conducts advocacy training seminars for such groups as the National Cancer Institute and to activists through the Centers for Disease Control and Prevention. This is from a training seminar conducted from November 6–8, 1991 for the National Cancer Institute's Project ASSIST: "ASSIST Training Materials, Volume 1, Orientation" (Bethesda, MD: Prospect Associates, December 3, 1991) pp. V-3,4.
2. CDC, Office on Smoking and Health, "National Tobacco Prevention and Control Program," 1994.
3. Ibid.
4. FDHRS proposal to CDC, awarded grant # U1A/CCU409238-01, September 15, 1993.
5. Ibid.
6. Ibid., p. 21.
7. Ibid.
8. Ibid., p. 59. See, also, Bennett and DiLorenzo, *CancerScam.*
9. Robert Wood Johnson Foundation, *Smokeless States: Statewide Tobacco Prevention and Control Initiatives 1996* (Princeton, NJ: RWJF, 1996).

10. Genevieve M. Young, "Robert Wood Johnson Foundation: One Philanthropy's Web of State Health Care Initiatives," *Organization Trends* (Washington, DC: Capital Research Center, August 1995).
11. Ibid., p. 5.
12. Ibid., p. 9.
13. STAT (Stop Teenage Addiction to Tobacco), "Getting Started with the STAT Campaign!" (STAT, 511 E Columbus Ave., Springfield, MA 01105).
14. Ibid., p. 12.
15. Ibid., p. 8.
16. Ibid., p. 11.
17. Ibid.
18. U.S. Department of Health and Human Services, Centers for Disease Control, *National Tobacco Prevention and Control Program, Progress Report*, Florida Dept. of Health and Rehabilitative Services, May 31, 1994.
19. Ibid.
20. Robert Wood Johnson Foundation, *Reducing Underage Drinking Through Community and State Coalitions* (Princeton, NJ: RWJF, 1996).
21. Ibid., p. 5.
22. See, also, Bennett and DiLorenzo, *CancerScam*.

# Chapter 7

1. *Action Alert* letter from APHA, May 27, 1993.
2. *The Nation's Health*, December 1993, p. 5.
3. Ibid., p. 16.
4. Ibid.
5. Ibid., p. 9.
6. Mary Corcoran, Roger Gordon, Deborah Loren, and Gary Solon, "The Association between Men's Economic Status and Their Family and Community Origins," *Journal of Human Resources* 27 (Fall 1992), pp. 575-601.
7. Ibid.
8. Renata Forste and Marta Tienda, "Race and Ethnic Variation in the Schooling Consequences of Female Adolescent Sexual Activity," *Social Science Quarterly* 73 (March 1992), pp. 12-30.
9. Mwangi S. Kimenyi, "Rational Choice, Culture of Poverty, and the Intergenerational Transmission of Welfare Dependency," *Southern Economic Journal* 57 (April 1991), pp. 947-60.
10. M. Anne Hill and June O'Neill, *Underclass Behaviors in the United States: Measurement and Analysis of Determinants* (New York: City University of New York, Baruch College, August 1993).
11. See, for example, Greg J. Duncan and Saul D. Hoffman, "Welfare Benefits, Economic Opportunities, and Out-of-Wedlock Births among Black Teenage Girls," *Demography* 27 (November 1990), pp. 519-35; and Robert Moffit, "Welfare Effects on Female Headship with Area Effects," *Journal of Human Resources* 29 (Spring 1994), pp. 621-36.
12. F.A. Peterson, J. Rubenstein, and L. Yarrow, "Infant Development in Father-Absent Families," *Journal of Genetic Psychology*, 135 (September 1979), pp. 51-61; J. Walsh, "Illegitimacy, Child-Abuse and Neglect, and Cognitive Development," *Journal of Genetic Psychology* 151 (September 1990), pp. 279-85.
13. Josefina J. Card, "Long-Term Consequences for Children of Teenage Parents," *Demography* 18 (May 1981), pp. 137-56.

14. Deborah Dawson, "Family Structure and Children's Health and Well-Being: Data from the 1988 National Health Interview Survey on Child Health," paper presented at the annual meeting of the Population Association of America, Toronto, Canada, May 1990.
15. D. Smith and G. Jarjoura, "Social Structure and Criminal Victimization," *Journal of Research in Crime and Delinquency* 25 (February 1988), pp. 27-52.
16. John Berlau, "EPA and FDA Put Ecology Above Kids," *Insight,* October 20, 1997, p. 14.
17. A thorough examination of this is found in Michael Fumento, *Polluted Science* (Washington, DC: AEI Press, 1997).
18. Peter Spencer, "Smog Control's Vanishing Returns," *Intellectual Capital.com* February 7, 1997.
19. Berlau, "EPA and FDA."
20. Ibid.
21. James T. Bennett and Thomas J. DiLorenzo, "The Commercialization of America's Health Charities," *Society* 34 (May/June 1997), pp. 67-72.
22. Special Section: APHA Annual Vote Tally, *The Nation's Health*, February 1997, pp. 8-16.
23. *The Nation's Health*, February 1997, p. 10.
24. Letters to the Editor, *The Nation's Health*, April 1996, p. 2.
25. Ibid.
26. "Reaffirming Affirmative Action," "President's Column," *The Nation's Health*, September 1995, p. 2.
27. Gail Herlot, "Doctored Affirmative-Action Data," *Wall Street Journal*, October 15, 1997.
28. Ibid.
29. Ibid.
30. Barry S. Levy, "Attacks on Proposed Clean-Air Standards Offer Lessons for All," *The Nation's Health*, July 1997, p. 2.
31. "Action Alert: Family Privacy Protection Act," *The Nation's Health*, June 1997.
32. Barry Levy, "PH Leadership 301: Student Case Study for the Year 2072," *The Nation's Health*, March 1997, p. 2.
33. Ibid.
34. E. Richard Brown, "A Public Health Agenda for Children," *The Nation's Health*, November 1996, p. 2.
35. U.S. Department of Commerce, *Statistical Abstract of the United States* (Washington, DC: U.S. Government Printing Office, 1997).
36. "With Stroke of Pen, Clinton Enacts APHA Choice Agenda, Zaps Quayle Council," *The Nation's Health*, February 1993, p. 1.
37. "Istook Amendment Would Curtail Lobbying by Non-Profit Groups," *The Nation's Health*, October 1995, p. 5.
38. *The Nation's Health*, March 1997, p. 9.
39. *The Nation's Health*, January 1995, p. 6.
40. *The Nation's Health*, October 1995, p. 4.
41. *The Nation's Health*, July 1997, p. 2.
42. *The Nation's Health*, September 1997, p. 11.

# Chapter 8

1. Joseph P. Martino, *Science Funding: Politics and Porkbarrel* (New Brunswick, NJ: Transaction Publishers, 1992).

## 150    From Pathology to Politics

2. Ibid., pp. 2-3.
3. Ibid., p. 4.
4. Edith Efron, *The Apocalyptics* (New York: Macmillan, 1984), pp. 433-34.
5. Ibid.
6. See Dixey Lee Ray, *Trashing the Planet* (Washington, DC: Regnery/Gateway, 1990), p. 83.
7. Ibid., p. 84.
8. Ibid., p. 85.
9. Robert Bidinotto, "The Great Apple Scare," *Readers Digest,* October 1990, p. 53.
10. For a lengthy discussion of the flaws in this research, see Sullum, *For Your Own Good.*
11. Steven Milloy, *Science Without Sense: The Risky Business of Public Health Research* (Washington, DC: Cato Institute, 1995).
12. Ibid., p. 2.
13. Ibid., p. 1.
14. Ibid., p. 5.
15. Ibid., p. 14.
16. Ibid.
17. Ibid., p. 28.
18. Ibid., p. 35.
19. Bennett and DiLorenzo, *CancerScam.*
20. Jacob Sullum, "Just How Bad Is Secondhand Smoke?" *National Review,* May 16, 1994, p. 51.
21. Sullum, *For Your Own Good*, p. 173.
22. Ibid.
23. Sullum, "Just How Bad," p. 52.
24. Ibid.
25. Michael Fumento, *Polluted Science: The EPA's Campaign to Expand Clean Air Regulations* (Washington, DC: American Enterprise Institute, 1997).
26. Ibid., p. 12.
27. Ibid., p. 10.
28. Ibid.
29. Ibid., pp. 11-12.
30. Ibid., p. 15.
31. Ibid., p. 18.
32. Ibid., pp. 20-21.
33. Laura Johannes, "Pollution Study Sparks Debate Over Secret Data," *Wall Street Journal*, April 1, 1997.
34. Lynn Payer, *Disease Mongers: How Doctors, Drug Companies, and Insurers Are Making You Feel Sick* (New York: John Wiley, 1992).
35. Michael K. Evans, "A Review of 'The Effect of Ordinances Requiring Smoke-Free Restaurants on Restaurant Sales' by Stanton A. Glantz and Lisa R.A. Smith," published by the Evans Group, March 1997.
36. Ibid., p. 15.
37. Peter Cummings, Thomas Koepsell, David Grosman, James Savarino, and Robert Thompson, "The Association between the Purchase of a Handgun and Homicide or Suicide," *American Journal of Public Health* 87 (June 1997), pp. 974-78.
38. Ibid., p. 974.
39. Antoine Messiah, Thierry Dart, Brenda Spencer, Josiane Warszawski, and the French National Survey on Sexual Behavior Group, "Condom Breakage and Slippage during Heterosexual Intercourse: A French National Survey."

40. Ibid., p. 421.
41. Ibid.
42. Ibid., p. 423.
43. Sally Guttmacher, Lisa Lieberman, David Ward, Nick Freudenberg, Alice Radosh, and Don Des Jarlais, "Condom Availability in New York City Public High Schools: Relationships to Condom Use and Sexual Behavior," *American Journal of Public Health* 87 (September 1997), pp. 1427-33.
44. Scott Burris, "The Invisibility of Public Health: Population-Level Measures in a Politics of Market Individualism," *American Journal of Public Health* 87 (December 1997), pp. 1607-10.
45. Helen Rodriquez-Trias, "Topics for Our Times: From Cairo to Beijing — Women's Agenda for Equality," *American Journal of Public Health* 86 (March 1996), pp. 305-06.
46. Helen Schauffler and John Wilkerson, "National health Care Reform and the 103rd Congress: The Activities and Influence of Public Health Advocates," *American Journal of Public Health,* 87 (July 1997), pp. 1107-12.

## Chapter 9

1. Jonathan B. Kotch, Craig H. Blakely, Sarah S. Brown, and Frank Y. Wong, eds., *A Pound of Prevention: The Case for Universal Maternity Care in the U.S.* (Washington, DC: American Public Health Association, 1992).
2. Ibid., p. xi.
3. Ibid., p. xii.
4. Ibid.
5. Ibid., p. xiii.
6. Ibid., p. xvi.
7. Ibid., p. xv.
8. Ibid., p. 9.
9. Ibid., p. 20.
10. Ibid., p. 23.
11. Ibid., p. 268.
12. Ibid., p. 258.
13. Ibid., p. 260.
14. Ibid.
15. Robert J. Samuelson, "Investing in Our Children," *Newsweek*, February 23, 1998, p. 45.
16. Ibid.
17. Ibid.
18. Ibid.
19. Ibid.
20. Pia Nordlinger, "ClintonCare II," *The Weekly Standard*, November 3, 1997, p. 17.
21. Ibid.
22. Maggie Gallagher, "Day Careless," *National Review*, January 26, 1998, p. 43.
23. Ibid., pp. 37-43.
24. Andrew Peyton Thomas, "A Dangerous Experiment in Child Rearing," *Wall Street Journal*, January 8, 1998.
25. Karl Zinsmeister, "The Problem with Day Care," *American Enterprise* (May/June 1998), p. 40.
26. Ibid., p. 41.

27. Cited in Darcy Olsen, "The Advancing Nanny State: Why the Government Should Stay Out of Child Care," Cato Institute *Policy Analysis* No. 285 (Washington DC: Cato Institute, October 23, 1997, p. 6.
28. Katherine Boo, "Most D.C. Day-Care Centers Have Expired Licenses," *Washington Post*, October 6, 1996.
29. Zinmeister, "The Problem with Day Care," p. 44.
30. Thomas D. Elias, "Defiant California Smokers Vow to Find Other Ways to Get Smokes," *Washington Times*, December 7, 1998.
31. California Children and Families First Initiative Constitutional Amendment and Statute, 1998, p. 1.
32. Ibid., p. 4.
33. Thomas Sowell, *Inside American Education: The Decline, The Deception, The Dogmas* (New York: Free Press, 1993), p. 35.
34. Ibid., p. 36.
35. Ibid., p. 38.
36. Ibid., p. 39.
37. Ibid., p. 43.
38. Ibid., p. 45.
39. Gary F. Kelly, *Learning About Sex: The Contemporary Guide for Young Adults* (New York: Barron's Educational Series, 1987), pp. 3-4.
40. Allan Carlson, "The Total Army Family," *Free Market*, June 1998, p. 1.
41. Ibid.
42. Ibid., p. 2.
43. Ibid.
44. Ibid.
45. Ibid., p. 3.
46. Allan Carlson, "The Military As an Engine of Social Change," in John Denson, ed., *The Costs of War: America's Pyrrhic Victories* (New Brunswick, NJ: Transaction Publishers, 1997), p. 331.

# Chapter 10

1. Robin Marantz Henig, *The People's Health:A Memoir of Public Health and Its Evolution at Harvard* (Washington, DC: Joseph Henry Press, 1997).
2. Ibid., inside back cover.
3. See Bennett and DiLorenzo, *Destroying Democracy*.
4. John R. Lott, Jr., *More Guns, Less Crime* (Chicago: University of Chicago Press, 1998).
5. C. Everett Koop, "The Link between Obesity and Disease," *Wall Street Journal*, Letters to the Editor, March 11, 1998.
6. Ibid.
7. Ibid.
8. Kelly D. Brownell, "Get Slim with Higher Taxes," *New York Times*, January 29, 1995.
9. Ibid.
10. Fredrich A. Hayek, *The Constitution of Liberty* (Chicago: University of Chicago Press, 1960), p. 71.

# Index

Lautenberg, Frank, 85
Levin, Carl, 92
Levinson, Sanford, 63
Levy, Barry S., 30, 87-88, 92
Lister, Joseph, 8
Little Mothers' Leagues, 11
Lobbying
    alcohol prohibitions, 73-74
    CDC and, 65
    children and, 70-71
    impact grants and, 66-69
    Johnson Foundation and, 69-70
    political progress and, 71-73
    tax dollars for, 65-66
*Lopez vs U. S.*, 18
Lott, John, 59, 138
Lyons, Joseph, 106

Malcolm, Joyce, 64
Martino, Joseph P., 96
Maryland Health Department, 15
Maternity care
    benefits of, 127-128
    civil service exemptions, 128
    competition eliminating, 128
    education on, 128
    goal of, 127
    government vs private, 119
    guideline establishing, 128-129
    nationalization of, 119, 127-129
    origin of, 127
    trust fund for, 120, 128
Media
    advocacy objectives, 54
    advocacy vs information, 53
    health defined in, 53
    vs individual choice, 54
Medicaid, cost of, 42
Medical savings accounts
    APHA and, 79
    benefits of, 79
    growth of, 80
    overview of, 79-80
    vs universal coverage, 80
Medicare, cost of, 42
Messick, Richard E., 31
Meyer, John G., 132
Milloy, Steve, 99-102, 108, 111
Moolgavkar, Suresh, 106
Moore, Stephen, 29
Moral-hazard problem

CCDP and, 122
    child care and, 118
    illegitimacy as, 82
Moyniham, Daniel Patrick, 78
Muray, Charles, 30
Musgrave, Gerald, 43

National Association for the Education
    of Young Children, 132
National Cancer Institute, 72, 98, 106
National Institutes of Health, 3, 17, 96
National Rifle Association, 60
National Science Board, 96
Nationalized health care
    child care into, 119-120
    funding for, 120-121
    insurance for, 38
    public policy and, 20
    record privacy in, 38
    vs private sector, 120
    *See also* Maternity care; Health care
        choice; Socialized health care
*Nation's Health*, 77, 85-86, 90
Nenno, Marcia, 68
Nestle Corporation, 51, 137
*New England Journal of Medicine*, 58,
    60, 109
New York Community Trust, 113
*New York Times*, 97, 107, 140
*Newsweek*, 122
Nicaraguan health care
    communist support of, 35-36
    conclusions on, 45
    expenditures of, 35-36
Nordlinger, Pia, 122
Nuclear Freeze Movement, 37

Obesity
    crisis of, 140
    political campaigns against, 140-141
    politicization of, 139-140
    premature deaths from, 140
O'Neill, June, 81

Partial birth abortion. *See* Abortion
Particulate matter
    EPA research on, 105-106
    lives saved from, 105
    opponent concerns vs, 107

local government grants, 23
profit motives, 32-34
public goods and, 21
reinventing of, 22-23
socialization in, 25-27
tax increase lobbying, 23
vs profit seeking, 33-34
vs traditional pursuits, 24
zero population growth, 27
Public health radicalization
bureaucracy and, 42-45
business, 51-52
economic policy pronouncements, 48-51
foreign policy, 35-37
risk analysis, 45-48
socializing health care, 37-42
Public health research
bias in, 95
content influencing, 96-97
funding of, 95
health risk exaggeration, 98
politician's career from, 98-99
politicization susceptibility, 95-96, 99-100
researcher competition, 97-98
special-interest politics in, 96
See also Risk assessments
Public Health Service (PHS)
gun control goals, 58
objectives of, 16-17
Public policy
APHA focus in, 19-20
national health insurance, 20

Quarantining
federal vs state in, 10-11
immigration and, 10-11
ships and, 10

Rather, Dan, 97
Richmond, Julius B., 135
Risk analysis
economic growth and, 48
EPA and, 47-48
essence of, 46
financial waste examples, 46-47
particulate matter and, 106
public health and, 45-46
"statistical murder" in, 46

study politics and, 138-139
Risk assessments
cancer cluster scares, 102
causation criteria, 100-101
data collection problems, 101-102
effectiveness misuse, 101
examples of, 100
health research politicization, 99-100
political science and, 99-102
public intuitive risks, 100
risk analysis relationships, 101
survey biases, 102
toxicology principles, 102
ubiquitous risks, 100
un-provable risks, 100
See also Public health research
Ritchie, Mark, 51
Robert Wood Johnson Foundation. See Johnson Foundation
Rodriguez-Trias, Helen, 114
Rossi, Peter, 59
Rozbicki, Mary-Ann, 44
Rubin, Robert, 122

Samuelson, Robert J., 122
Satel, Sally, 25-26, 28, 30
Schaffer, Henry E., 59
Schid, Frederick, 68
Schuman, Stanley, 124
Second Amendment
CDC studies, 62
public health and, 137-138
rights under, 57-58
support for, 63-64
vs "new" rights, 63
See also Gun Control
Second hand smoke
EPA and, 99-103
epidemiological studies, 103-105
health risk of, 103
research credibility, 103
Sex education, 129-130
Sims, Joyner, 67
Smith, Adam, 122
Social Security Act, 17
Socialized health care
beneficiaries of, 42
budget spending, 40-41
capital expenditures, 44-45
caring vs curing, 44
central planning of, 37-38

Printed in the United States
by Baker & Taylor Publisher Services